DRUGS AND BEHAVIOR:

A Primer in
Neuropsychopharmacology

ERNEST L. ABEL

Research Institute on Alcoholism
Buffalo, New York

A WILEY-INTERSCIENCE PUBLICATION

JOHN WILEY & SONS

New York   London   Sydney   Toronto

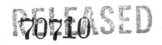

Library of Congress Cataloging in Publication Data:

Abel, Ernest L   1943-
  Drugs and behavior.

  "A Wiley-Interscience publication."
  Bibliography: p.
  1. Neuropsychopharmacology. I. Title.
[DNLM: 1. Psychopharmacology. QV77 A139d]

RM315.A22   615'.78   74-8969
ISBN 0-471-00155-4

Printed in the United States of America

10 9 8 7 6 5 4 3 2 1

Preface

This book has been written for those students who need or simply desire more than a cursory overview of the principles of neuropharmacology, but who do not have the time, background, or inclination to master the more formidible textbooks in this area. Those whose main interest is in the behavioral aspects of drug action will probably derive the greatest use from this material, since I have tried to provide the reader both with a better understanding of the mechanisms of drug action and with a better appreciation of the ways in which drugs can be used to elucidate the mechanisms' underlying behavior.

To understand how drugs affect behavior, it is important to know something about the way in which the mechanisms' underlying behavior operates. This involves a consideration of cellular functioning as well as a passing familiarity with the functional organization of cells in the central nervous system. In this regard, it is also important to know something about the movement of drugs from their sites of administration to their cellular sites of action and the transformations to which they are subjected during this movement. This, in essence, is the structure around which the discussion of drug action revolves.

It is possible, of course, to disregard mechanisms of drug action and problems of absorption, distribution, metabolism, etc., and to concentrate solely on a strict stimulus-response approach. This, however, ignores the fact that organisms are biological entities. Between the chemical stimulus and the behavioral response are physiological changes that directly or indirectly mediate empirical stimulus-response effects. Without a knowledge of the principles involved in drug action there can be no real understanding of the ways in which drugs affect behavior; there can only be a collection of individual facts.

In dealing with this subject, I have tried to present the material in the context of well-known biological principles. However, because of obvious space limitation, I have had both to simplify and to be selective in my choice of this material. Those who desire more information concerning a particular problem or topic would do well to consult the original papers alluded to in the discussion. Hopefully, this book will inform the reader. If it should also possibly stimulate him to inquire further into the many potentialities for using drugs to investigate the chemical basis of behavior, then this book will have realized the purpose for which it was intended.

ERNEST L. ABEL

Buffalo, New York
April 1974

Acknowledgments

A work of this nature recognizably involves assistance, advice, and encouragement from many individuals. Among those to whom special appreciation is extended are my colleague Dr. A. J. Siemens of the Research Institute on Alcoholism, whose comments have been of great value, and my wife Barbara, who followed the progress of the text with interest and encouragement. Special appreciation is extended also to the various authors and publishers who allowed me to incorporate material from their publications into my own. These publications and publishers are acknowledged gratefully in the list that follows.

From Miller, N., Gottesman, K., and Emery, N., *American Journal of Physiology,* **206**: 1384–1388, 1964, figure 6; From Grossman, S. P., *ibid.,* **202**: 872–882, 1962, figures 1 and 4; **202**: 1230–1236, 1962, figures 2 and 5.

From Brodie, B. B., in Binns, T. B. (Ed.), *Absorption and Distribution of Drugs,* 1964, figure 1, p. 201. Courtesy of Churchill Livingstone, Edinburgh.

From Calesnick, B., in DiPalma, J. R. (Ed.), *Drill's Pharmacology,* 1965, figure 6-3. Courtesy of McGraw-Hill, New York.

From Elliott, H. C., *Textbook of Neuroanatomy,* figure 2-3, 1969. Courtesy of J. P. Lippincott, Philadelphia.

From Faulconer, A., and Bickford, R. G., *Electroencephalography In Anesthesiology,* 1960, figure 4. Courtesy of Charles C Thomas, Springfield, Ill.

From Loomis, T. A., *Essentials of Toxicology,* 1968, figure 3-1. Courtesy of Lea and Febiger, Philadelphia.

From Jasper, H. H., in Penfield, W., and Erickson, T. C. (Eds.) *Epilepsy and Cerebral Localization,* 1941, figure 121. Courtesy of Charles C Thomas, Springfield, Ill.

From Toner, P. G., and Carr, K. E., *Cell Structure*, 1960, figure 1. Courtesy of Williams and Wilkins, Baltimore.

From Stevens, C. F., *Neurophysiology: A Primer*, 1966, figure 1-1. Courtesy of John Wiley, New York.

From Daniels, T. C., and Jorgensen, O., in Wilson, C. O., Gisvold, O., and Doerge, R. F. (Eds.), *Textbook of Organic Medicinal and Pharmaceutical Chemistry*, 1971, p. 33. Courtesy of J. P. Lippincott, Philadelphia.

From *American Journal of Physiology,* **206**: 1384–1388, 1964, figure 6; **202**: 872–882, 1962, figures 1 and 4; **202**: 1230–1236, 1962, figures 2 and 5.

From Barnett, A., Goldstein, J., and Taber, R. I., *Archives Internationales de Pharmacodynamie*, **198**: 242–247, 1972, figure 2.

From Warner, G. F., Dobson, E. L., and Pace, N., *Circulation*, **8**: 732–734, 1953, figure 1. Courtesy of The American Heart Association, Inc.

From Schuster, C. R., *Federation Proceedings*, **29**: 2–5, 1970, figure 2.

From De Robertis, E. D. D., *International Review of Cytology*, **8**: 61–95, 1959, figure 1. Courtesy of Academic Press, New York.

From Starzl, T. E., Taylor, C. W., and Magoun, H. W., *Journal of Neurophysiology*, **14**: 461–496, 1951, figure 8.

From Goldberg, N. D., and Shideman, F. E., *Journal of Pharmacology and Experimental Therapeutics,* **136**: 142–151, 1962, figure 3; From Reis, D. J., Corvelli, A., and Connors, J. *ibid.,* **167**: 328–333, 1969, figure 2. Courtesy of Williams and Wilkins, Baltimore.

From Grossman, S. P., *Science*, **132**: 301–302, July 1960, figure 2. Courtesy of the American Association for the Advancement of Science.

ERNEST L. ABEL

Contents

Contents   ix

1. The Structural and Functional Basis of Behavior

THE CHARACTERISTICS OF LIFE

The fundamental unit of all living organisms, regardless of their complexity, is the cell. Because they are incapable of defining what life is, however, biologists have found it expedient to describe the essential characteristics of living things on the basis of properties that can be measured either directly or indirectly. Accordingly, organisms are said to be alive if they possess the following traits.

1. A specific structural and chemical organization.
2. The ability to take in food and to release the potential energy contained therein for purposes of doing work (metabolism).
3. The capacity to make new cellular components from the simple products into which food has been broken down (growth and repair).
4. The ability to eliminate by-products of metabolism (elimination).
5. The capacity to respond to stimulation (irritability).
6. The ability to move (contractability).
7. The ability to reproduce.

Although some organisms that do not possess all these characteristics are still considered to be "alive," the vast majority of living organisms are capable of performing each and every one of these functions.

The organizational characteristics of living organisms can be examined from several different viewpoints. For example, even the most elementary forms of life, such as the single-celled organisms (e.g., the amoeba and the paramecium), are characterized by each of these features. Even these creatures can be broken down into more fundamental units such as the molecule and the atom, but atoms and molecules by themselves are not considered to be "living" since they do not possess all the basic characteristics listed above. When groups of different molecules come together in a certain organization, on the other hand, a cell such as the amoeba may be formed which can be identified as living on the basis of the aforementioned criteria.

At the next level of complexity, one may examine how cells of similar types unite to form tissues. For example, muscle tissue is composed of muscle cells. Different tissues may then be organized into organs such as the heart and the kidney, which in turn are organized into systems. For example, the cardiovascular system has emerged as the mechanism responsible for distributing food, oxygen, and the products of metabolism to the various cells of the bodies of multicellular organisms.

At still another level, it is possible to study how the cardiovascular system along with the other systems, for example, respiratory and reproductive, are organized in a way that enables a complex multicellular organism to function as a living unit. The most complex organism can thus be regarded as essentially a collection of cells.

Since in the final analysis most drug activity results from the action of drugs on individual cells, this first chapter is devoted to a more detailed consideration of some of the important structures and functions that are characteristic of these basic units of life.

THE STRUCTURE OF CELLS

Despite gross differences in size, shape, and functions, all cells are basically similar in that they possess an outer membrane within which are contained cytoplasm and a nucleus. A highly schematic representation of a hypothetical cell is depicted in Fig. 1.1.

Cellular membranes are composed almost entirely of protein and lipid (fat) material. The exact molecular organization of the cell membrane is not known for certain as yet, but there is a great deal of evidence pointing to a structure such as that depicted in the model shown in Fig. 1.2. As reflected in this diagram, cellular membranes are thought to be composed of a double layer of lipids (fats) surrounded on either side by a layer of protein. This lipoprotein structure has important implications for the activity by limiting the passage of lipid-insoluble substances into the interior of the cell. The passage of positively and negatively charged ions across the cell membrane also is limited as a consequence of this structural peculiarity. This means that some cells may have a much higher proportion of positive or negative ions outside the membrane relative to the interior. Such membranes are said to be polarized.

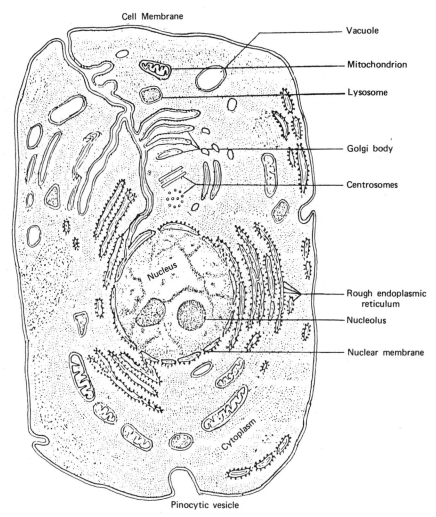

Fig. 1.1   Schematic diagram of a cell.

Although they have never been observed even with electron microscopes, experimental evidence suggests that membranes also contain minute pores which allow very small molecular substances to flow into and out of the cell. It is through such pores that lipid-insoluble substances such as water are able to move into and out of cells with relative ease. It is also thought that in some specialized cells, such as those involving the transmission of neural impulses, these pores are capable of enlarging, thereby permitting the entry of ions that previously were unable to enter the cell because of their size.

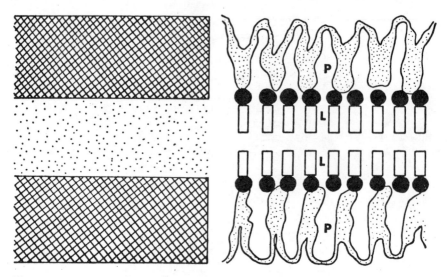

Fig. 1.2 Model of cell membrane structure. On the left is a representative of the trilaminar appearance of a biological membrane as seen by transmission electron microscopy. The two external dense laminae are separated by a pale interspace. On the right is a possible molecular interpretation of this membrane structure. The double layer of lipid molecules, L, is surrounded on either side by a layer of protein, P. The black circles represent hydrophilic polar components of the lipid molecules which are believed to be associated with the protein component of the membrane (from Toner and Carr, 1968).

One well-known drug whose pharmacological activity is based almost solely on its ability to disrupt the integrity of bacterial cell walls is the antibiotic penicillin. By preventing the synthesis of new cell walls in certain bacteria that cause disease, penicillin essentially prevents them from existing as an entity. The reason that penicillin is not toxic to mammalian cells is because these cells lack a material in their cell walls which is unique to the bacteria, and which is the part of the wall that attracts penicillin and thereby leads to its own destruction.

The bulk of the cell interior is cytoplasm, which consists of about 60 to 90% water, with the rest being electrolytes, proteins, lipids, carbohydrates, and organelles. This high water content enables water-soluble materials to be distributed evenly throughout the cell and facilitates chemical interaction between water-soluble elements. The main electrolytes found in cells are potassium, magnesium, calcium, phosphate, chloride, bicarbonate, and sodium. The electrolytes serve many functions, some of which are described in detail in this chapter. Protein is made up of small molecular substances called amino acids, and provides the structural framework of the interior of the cell and its membranes. Protein also provides the enzymes essential for processes such as nerve conduction, muscle contraction, and metabolism that take place in cells. Lipids are fatty substances that act in conjunction with protein in forming the cell membrane as well as the nuclear and organelle membranes. The carbohydrate content of the cell acts as an energy reservoir which is necessary if the cell is to function properly in emergency situations. Most of the carbohydrate in the interior of a cell is stored as glycogen, an insoluble form of glucose.

The remaining constituents of the cytoplasm are physical structures called organelles (little organs). The main organelles are the endoplasmic reticulum, ribosomes, nucleus, mitochondria, and lysosomes. Together they take care of the growth and maintenance of the cell. Since the effects of many drugs are related directly to their influence on the activity of these organelles, the structure and function of these bodies are described in somewhat greater detail than was devoted to the other fractions of the cytoplasm.

The endoplasmic reticulum as depicted in Fig. 1.1 is a lacelike network consisting essentially of pairs of membranes which enclose an interconnecting series of cavities called cisternae. Actually, there are two main types of endoplasmic reticulum, designated rough (granular) or smooth (agranular) on the basis of their appearance.

One of the main functions of this structure is the metabolism and detoxication of materials that are foreign to the interior of the cell. Various enzyme systems, apparently present for just this purpose, appear to be associated with the surface of the endoplasmic reticulum; by means of the interconnecting network of cisternae, they are provided with the materials which enable them to inactivate substances that might otherwise be a danger to the integrity of the cell.

Ribosomes are small particles, some of which move about freely in the cytoplasm and some of which are attached to the outer surface of the endoplasmic reticulum, thus accounting for its granular appearance. These small bodies are made up largely of ribonucleic acid (RNA) and constitute the site of protein synthesis in the cell. This protein producing function is controlled by the genetic code associated with desoxyribonucleic acid (DNA) which is contained in the cell nucleus. The "instructions" from nuclear DNA to ribosomal RNA for the manufacture of protein are mediated by a kind of RNA called "messenger" RNA (mRNA). The group of antibiotic drugs that go by the name of streptomycin derive their main ability to fight bacterial infection as a result of interfering with the sending of these messages from DNA to the ribosomes. By preventing the attachment of messenger RNA to its ribosomes in bacterial cells, streptomycin essentially blocks or distorts the message coming to the ribosome.

As a result, either the protein material formed by the bacteria is abnormal, or the amount produced is below the level needed for continued functioning.

The energy requirements of the cell are looked after by the mitochondria. Under the microscope, mitochondria appear as a series of fine inner membranes surrounded by an outer membrane which keeps them intact. The interiors of these mitochondria contain oxidative enzymes which catalyze the formation of adenosine triphosphate (ATP) from glucose, phosphate ions, and adenosine diphosphate (ADP) by a process called oxidative phosphorylation.

The actual process by which energy is made available to the cell involves the transfer of electrons from glucose to ATP during several stages of oxidation and reduction. Oxidation refers to the removal of electrons from atoms or molecules; reduction denotes the addition of electrons. In the cell, these two reactions usually amount to the removal or addition of hydrogen atoms since hydrogen is nearly always involved.

Among the main compounds involved in the oxidation-reduction reaction are a number of molecules located in the mitochondria called the cytochromes. These cytochromes are designated b, c, a, a_3 (also called cytochrome oxidase), etc. Regardless of type, each of these cytochromes contains a single atom of iron in its structure which can exist in the ferrous (Fe^{2+}) or the ferric (Fe^{3+}) condition. In the ferrous state, the cytochrome molecule is in a reduced condition, whereas in the ferric state it is oxidized. Thus when electrons pass from ferric cytochrome b to ferrous cytochome c, the former is oxidized to ferrous cytochrome b whereas the latter is reduced to ferric cytochrome c. These cytochrome transfers, however, are only the intermediary steps in the energy transfer system. The initial electron acceptors are nicotinamide adenine dinucleotide (NAD), nicotinamide adenine phosphate (NADP), and flavin adenine dinucleotide (FAD). The nicotinamides are some of the initial hydrogen acceptors, whereas FAD usually acts to transfer electrons from NAD and NADP to the cytochromes.

The process begins with the removal of two hydrogen atoms from a substrate such as glucose, by NAD under the influence of a dehydrogenase enzyme. The hydrogens are transferred to FAD and then through the cytochrome chain and are finally passed by cytochrome oxidase to oxygen to form H_2O. During this transfer process, energy is generated from the oxidation reactions; this energy is used to produce high energy phosphate bonds in ATP from ADP and inorganic phosphate at various sites in the oxidative chain (see Fig. 1.3).

The basis for the increased store of energy in ATP results from a unique rearrangement of electrons that are shared by the phosphorus and oxygen atoms in the molecule. Both high and low energy phosphate bonds contain

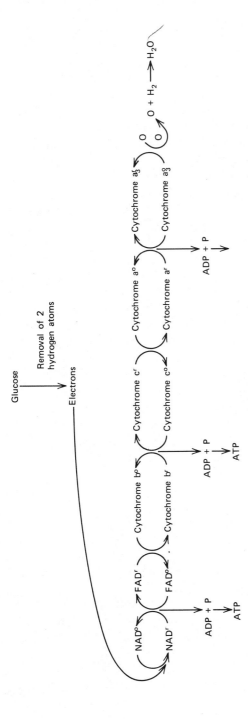

Fig. 1.3 Schematic representation of steps in passage of electrons during formation of ATP. During transfer, energy from electrons is used to add inorganic phosphate (P) to ADP to produce ATP. At the final step, electrons are passed by cytochrome oxidase (a_3) to molecular oxygen to form water. Superscripts: o, oxidized, r, reduced.

the same number of these atoms, but because of the unique atomic con-figurations associated with ATP, more energy is released when these bonds are broken than occurs in the case of other compounds. For example, high energy bonds release about 10 kcal compared with only 2 to 3 kcal for low energy bonds.

Each ATP molecule contains two of these "high energy" bonds which, when split, release a large amount of energy to all parts of the cell. This energy is used to transport substances such as sodium and potassium across their concentration gradients during the transmission of nerve impulses. It also provides the energy required for the mechanical work of the cell such as contraction, and for the synthesis of substances such as protein that are necessary for the maintenance of the cell. Without the energy provided by ATP, almost all the activities which organisms are capable of performing simply would not occur.

Interference with this mechanism would thus have obvious effects, and indeed, there is a great deal of experimental evidence indicating that many of the drugs that depress neural activity in the central nervous system (CNS) do so by interfering with the oxidative processes by which the brain derives almost all of its energy (cf. Quastel, 1967). For instance, cyanide causes death by combining with the last cytochrome in the electron transfer process and thereby completely inhibits its activity. As a result, oxygen can no longer reoxidize the cytochromes so that the initial carriers, NAD and FAD, cannot be reoxidized as they are during the normal process of oxidation and energy production. Hence the cells are deprived of their energy and die. Another drug, 2,4-dinitrophenol acts to prevent the forma-tion of high energy phosphate bonds; although oxidation still occurs, the process of oxidative phosphorylation is "uncoupled" and so energy produc-tion is curtailed.

The final organelle to be discussed is the lysosome. Lysosomes appear as dense particles in various areas of the cytoplasm and are responsible for the digestive functions of the cell. When these particles come into contact with foreign food-protein materials, they engulf them, much as the amoeba engulfs food. Digestive enzymes then break these food proteins down into amino acids, which subsequently are released back into the cell for pur-poses of reconversion into other protein material.

The digestive enzymes contained in these lysosomes are rather indis-criminate in their substrates, and if they were to escape from the interior of the lysosome, they would digest all the protein material of the cell, re-sulting in its eventual death. This in fact sometimes happens when the cells of the body are overexposed to radiation. It has also been suggested that rupture of the lysosomal membrane may be a factor in the etiology of certain diseases such as cancer.

There are a number of other organelles present in the cytoplasm such as the Golgi apparatus, centrosomes, and inclusions. Information regarding the function of these bodies may be found in texts dealing specifically with cell biology and are not commented upon here.

The third major feature in the morphology of the cell is the nucleus. The interior of the nucleus is composed primarily of nucleoplasm, DNA, and RNA (the nucleolus). Nucleoplasm has much the same function as cytoplasm; that is, it facilitates chemical movement and interaction within the nucleus. The genetic information that determines the structure and function of each cell is contained in the DNA. The process by which DNA exerts its influence is by dictating the kinds of protein and enzymes that the cell manufactures. This influence is essential for the continued existence of the cell since without the nucleus, the cell is unable to survive longer than a few days at most. The other main component of the nucleus is an aggregation of loosely bound granules which are referred to collectively as the nucleolus. These granular bodies are made up largely of RNA and are believed to be involved in the communication of instructions from DNA to cytoplasmic organelles such as the ribosomes. In addition to the fluids they contain, the cells of the body are surrounded by extracellular fluids from which they are able to take up oxygen and nutrients and into which they are able to discharge waste material. The extracellular fluid itself is divided into two components, the blood and the interstitial fluid. The blood is made up of plasma and certain bodies such as red blood cells. The interstitial fluid lies outside the cell and is separated from the blood by the capillary wall. This wall permits the free movement of water and minute particles from the blood to the interstitial fluid but prevents the movement of plasma proteins and other components of the blood from similar activity.

CELLULAR DIFFERENTIATION

Although basically similar with respect to their nuclear-cytoplasmic organization, living cells are also characterized by a remarkable diversity of form and function. However, neither of these two cellular features can account for the difference between a man and a mouse. The essential distinction between any two species lies rather in the organizational complexity of their cellular groups. When heart, muscle, or brain cells are removed from an organism and are placed in a nutrient bath, they rhythmically twitch, contract, display irritability, etc., but they do not constitute a heart, a muscle, or a brain. The differnce between cells growing in vitro, even thousands of cells, and those growing in the body (in vivo) lies not on the morphological and functional but the organizational level.

In single-celled organisms, the protozoa, all the functions necessary for life take place in the one cell. Single-celled animals have evolved even to the extent that they display sensitivity to external stimuli such as light, heat, and chemicals and are able to respond to such stimulation by approach and avoidance movements.

The circumstances that originally caused cells to aggregate are unknown, but the result of such aggregation was the emergence of multicellular organisms, the Metazoa. By working in conjunction with one another, individual cells now had a greater possibility for specialization and a division of labor between them. This in turn meant an increased opportunity for efficient organization and consequently a greater potential for complexity of behavior. The price of this increase in efficiency and complexity, however, was a relative loss of functional independence by each of the component members of the multicellular complex. For example, red blood cells have become so specialized that they no longer possess a nucleus and are essentially little more than packets of hemoglobin that carry oxygen to the various cells of the body. Liver cells, on the other hand, have specialized in enzymatic activity with resultant changes in the endoplasmic reticulum found in their cytoplasm. As a consequence of its enzymatic activity, the liver has emerged as the main site for the metabolic inactivation of drugs in the body.

The most highly organized aggregation of cells known to man is found in his own human nervous system. This consists of the brain and the spinal cord, which together are referred to as the central nervous system (CNS), and the nework of nerves that connect them with all the other parts of the body, the peripheral nervous system (PNS). The CNS not only serves as the communication link between receptor (sensory) and effector (motor) organs, but also integrates the information it receives and on the basis of this information makes "decisions" that enable the organism to modify its behavior. A branch of the peripheral nervous system that bears special mention is called the autonomic nervous system (ANS). This system is involved in the maintenance of a stable internal physiological environment (homeostasis). As such, it regulates the functioning of various internal organs and glands such as the heart, the liver, and the genitals.

The overall structural and functional characteristics of cells have been discussed at some length, because to understand how drugs are capable of influencing the behavior of an organism, it is necessary to examine the substrates upon which drugs act. Familiarity with the structure and functions of cells is important therefore, because it provides an insight into the many potential ways by which drugs can affect the integrity of an organism. It is with this point in mind that we now pass on to a more detailed examination of the structure and functions of a particular cell, the neuron.

STRUCTURE OF THE NEURON

The functional unit of the nervous system is the nerve cell or neuron. Regardless of size or appearance, each neuron basically consists of a cell body and its attendant processes, the dendrites and axon. The dendrites are the receiving part of the neuron and they conduct impulses from other neurons to the cell body, although the cell body may receive impulses directly from other neurons as well. Actually, dendrites are nothing more than direct extensions of the cell body and as such they contain mitochondria and Nissl bodies (see below). The axon is the part of the neuron that carries impulses away from the cell body to other neurons or to effector organs such as muscles and glands. Although an axon may give off collateral branches, the main branching occurs at its end where it terminates into many telodendria, which are buttonlike structures called by various terms such as terminal buttons, synaptic boutons, and end feet. Actual and schematic representations of one kind of neuron are shown in Fig. 1.4.

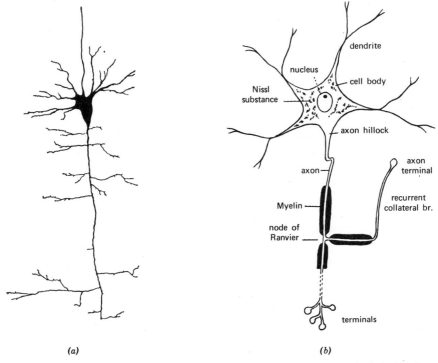

(a)   (b)

Fig. 1.4 Actual and schematic appearance of a neuron (a) A typical multipolar neuron from the motor cortex as it appears when treated with a special staining material (Nissl stain). (b) Schematic depiction of a generalized multipolar neuron (from Elliott, 1972, and Everett, 1971).

The various types of nerve cells are classified on the basis of the number and pattern of processes arising from the cell body. The first is the unipolar neuron, so named because it has only one process which functions both as dendrite and as axon to receive and transmit information. The second type is the bipolar neuron. This has a distinct dendrite and a distinct axon. The single dendrite often divides into numerous smaller branches, each of which may receive information from other neurons. The final type of neuron is the multipolar cell. This has one axon but several dendrites, each of which, by branching, is able to collect information from an incredible number of other neurons.

The cell body (also called the soma or perikaryon) contains the same organelles and performs the same functions that have been discussed previously with reference to cells in general. In addition to these organelles, nerve cells possess another type of structure called Nissl bodies, which are quite prominent in the cytoplasm of the nerve cell body. The function of these Nissl bodies is still quite conjectural, although the state of the neuron tends to be intimately linked with the state of the Nissl bodies. For instance, during chronic stimulation of nerve cells, the Nissl bodies become depleted of their contents. Injury to the nerve cell also affects these organelles, resulting in a condition called chromatolysis (loss of Nissl substance).

The axon and the nerve impulse both arise from an area associated with the cell body called the axon hillock. However, the axon hillock does not seem to be an actual part of the cell body since it does not contain any Nissl bodies. This is also true of the axon. Some axons, however, do possess a distinctive feature of their own called myelin, which surrounds them and acts as an insulator, thereby facilitating the conduction of impulses. This myelin covering is not continuous, however, but is periodically interrupted by what are referred to as nodes of Ranvier. These too have a facilitating effect on nerve conduction.

The size and length of the nerve axon generally reflect the efficiency and the function of a particular cell. For instance, axons that have large diameters are able to conduct impulses much more rapidly than those with smaller diameters. In addition the axons of some neurons, such as those found in the peripheral nervous system, may be as long as several feet and are known as Golgi type I neurons. The main function of these cells is to transmit information from sensory receptors to the brain and to carry "instructions" from the brain to effector organs. Nerve cells that have short axons are known as Golgi type II neurons and are characteristic of the interneuronal cells of the brain which are responsible for the integration and processing of all the information available to the organism.

Between the synaptic boutons of one neuron and the dendrites of another is a minute cleft called the synapse. Impulses are not transmitted directly across this cleft; instead, a chemical is released from the pre-synaptic area which diffuses across the cleft and then causes an impulse to be initiated in the postsynaptic membrane. With the aid of the electron microscope, tiny vesiclelike structures have been identified in the synaptic bouton. It is believed that these morphological structures contain the chemicals which mediate transmission from neuron to neuron, or from neuron to muscle or to other effector organs (e.g., glands). The structure of the synaptic bouton is discussed at greater length later in this chapter.

The principal difference between the brain of man and that of any other species is not due to his possessing any particular kind of neuron that differs from those of other species. The structures just described are found in both man and subhumans. As noted earlier, the difference lies rather in the incredible organizational complexity of the neurons in the human brain.

Although Fig. 1.5 gives only a simplified representation of what this complexity is really like, it does make the point readily apparent that it is simply not possible to comprehend the activity of the CNS in terms of the workings and interrelation of only a few isolated neurons. Nevertheless, discovering the way in which a few isolated neurons function is a first step toward understanding how larger groups of nerve cells may act upon one another to produce the complex phenomenon that is behavior.

THE RESTING AND ACTION POTENTIALS

Nerve fibers consist of groups of neurons that are held together by connective tissue. Whereas a neuron is an individual nerve cell, a nerve trunk, or nerve, is essentially made up of hundreds or thousands of axons, each arising from a separate neuronal cell body. If a small electrode is inserted into the interior of a nerve fiber and is then connected through a voltmeter to another electrode located outside the fiber, a small electrical potential difference of about -60 to -70 mV, called the resting potential, is observed. Instead of a voltmeter, however, potential differences in nerves are more commonly measured by means of an oscilloscope. With this instrument, it is possible to amplify the changes in potential so that they can be measured with greater precision. This allows the almost instantaneous detection of very small changes in the resting potential.

The term electrical potential refers to any situation in which there is an uneven distribution of electrically charged particles between any two points. In the case of a neuron, an electrical potential exists between the interior and exterior of the cell because the cell membrane is permeable to some ions but not to others. Although the number of different ions associated with nerve cells is considerable (e.g., Na^+, Cl^-, K^+ Ca^{2+}, Mg^{2+}, and HCO_3^-), the two principal ions that account for the transmembrane resting

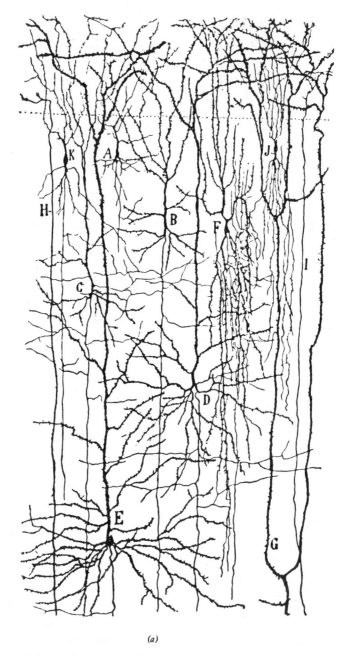

(a)

Fig. 1.5a Various neurons from the frontal cortex of a 1-month-old child are depicted as they appear in a preparation of nerve tissue that has been treated to bring out these features (Golgi preparation) (Ramon y Cajal, 1911).

14

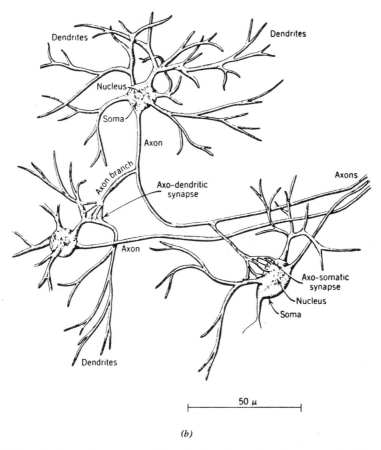

(b)

Fig. 1.5*b*   A schematic representation of three interrelated neurons depicting the anatomical features of each cell (Stevens, 1966).

potential and the electrical activity of the cell are potassium and sodium. The intracellular and extracellular distribution of these two ions is shown in Table 1.1.

As indicated by the table, there is about 30 times more intracellular K^+ than outside the cell. Conversely, there is about 12 times more extracellular Na^+ relative to the interior.

The explanation for the resting potential is thought to result from the relative permeabilities of the nerve cell membrane to postassium and sodium ions. At rest, the membrane is slightly permeable to potassium ions and because of the concentration gradient, these ions move out of the axon. But as they leave the axon, they create an increase in negativity within the axon owing to the excess of negative ions that remain behind.

Table 1.1 Intra- and Extracellular Distribution of
Sodium and Potassium Ions (Approximate)

Ion	Intracellular (meq /liter	Extracellular (meq /liter)
Potassium	150	5
Sodium	12	145

The increase in negativity within the axon now begins to attract the positively charged potassium ions back across the membrane until at about -75 mV, an equilibrium potassium potential is achieved at which the rate of potassium ions leaving the axon is equal to that of potassium ions moving into the axon.

In the case of sodium ions, the opposite happens. With an axonal concentration of sodium ions far below that outside the membrane, sodium ions would tend to move into the cell owing to the concentration gradient. However, when the membrane is at rest the hydrated sodium ion, which is much larger than the hydrated potassium ion, is not able to pass through the membrane pores to any great extent. As a result there is hardly any net movement of sodium ions into the axon. Contrariwise, hydrated potassium ions are smaller than hydrated sodium ions and are therefore able to traverse the nerve cell membrane much more easily.

The potential of the resting nerve cell can thus be regarded as being due almost entirely to the differential distribution of potassium ions across the nerve cell membrane. Since this membrane potential eventually disappears from cells that are deprived of oxygen, it appears that there is an active mechanism responsible for the maintenance of the membrane potential and that this mechanism is dependent upon metabolic processes such as those involved in oxidative phosphorylation as outlined above. Thus drugs that affect the access of oxygen to nerve cells have the effect of diminishing the resting nerve cell potential. As will be seen in a moment, this has the effect of preventing the conduction of nerve impulses.

Nerve impulses, termed action potentials, are initiated when there is a change in the cell membrane so that sodium ions are no longer prevented from entering the cell. Since ions flow in the direction of high to low concentrations, sodium ions begin to rush into the cell. This not only abolishes the resting potential, but actually drives it in the opposite direction. At the same time, however, potassium ions start to rush out from the interior since the electrical potential holding them back has been diminished by the movement of sodium ions. This outward movement of potassium acts to oppose somewhat the electrical effect of the inward moving sodium ions.

The influx of sodium, however, is so much greater than the efflux of potassium that the interior of the cell becomes slightly positive by about 40 mV. This change, called a depolarization, lasts for only a brief instant. The membrane then returns to its previous permeability characteristics in which sodium is again prevented from entering the cell. In addition, the cell begins actively to secrete the sodium ions that became trapped in the interior.

Once one area of the cell membrane becomes depolarized, however, the influx of sodium ions into that area causes adjacent regions of the membrane to become more permeable to sodium ions as well. This alteration in the resting potential is passed on down the neuron until it either reaches the synaptic boutons or encounters a region of the cell membrane which has been treated with some agent (e.g., a local anesthetic) that prohibits any further change in membrane permeability.

The movement of sodium ions out of the cell after the peak of the action potential can be demonstrated by "loading" the relatively large squid axon with radioactively labeled sodium ions. This is done by stimulating the nerve while it is immersed in a bath of seawater containing radioactive sodium. If the axon is then washed continuously with seawater containing ordinary sodium ions and this fluid is collected and properly analyzed, it is found to contain radioactivity that could come from no other source than the sodium ions that have been trapped and then expelled from the cell (Hodgkin, 1958).

The fact that the extrusion of sodium involves an active metabolic process was demonstrated by exposing axons to 2,4-dinitrophenol (DNP). One of the major effects of this compound is that it interferes with oxidative phosphorylation (see above). Consequently the addition of DNP prevents the efflux of Na^+ from the axon since there is no longer any energy source to drive the "sodium pump" (see Fig. 1.6). The results of experiments such as these provide additional proof that the mechanism responsible for keeping sodium ions out of the cell involves energy. Further evidence for this hypothesis is the finding that injections of ATP directly into the axon restore its ability to extrude sodium (Hodgkin and Keynes, 1955).

THE CONCEPT OF THRESHOLD

The strength of the stimulus just sufficient to produce an action potential is referred to as the threshold intensity. However, the magnitude of this threshold stimulus is not constant but varies as a function of its time characteristics as well as its intensity. For instance, if a subthreshold stimulus is applied to an axon for a relatively long time, the membrane becomes fully charged and the threshold strength of the stimulus required to pro-

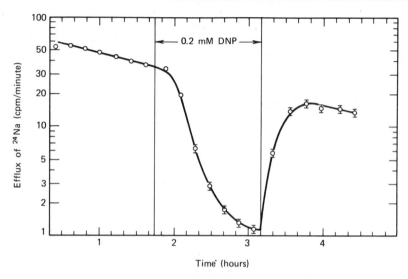

Fig. 1.6   Effect of 2,4-dinitrophenol (DNP) on sodium efflux from nerve axons. The axon was first stimulated in seawater containing radioactively labeled sodium (^{24}Na). The axon was then placed in an apparatus in which fluid could be drawn past the axon and collected. The seawater was then replaced with a similar solution containing DNP. After about 10 minutes the efflux of sodium was reduced to about 1/20 of the previous rate. When the DNP was removed from the seawater, this inhibitory effect was reversed (modified from Hodgkins and Keynes, 1955).

duce an action potential is less than that for a brief stimulus. Consequently, in examining the conduction properties of nerves, neurophysiologists take into consideration not only the intensity but also the duration of the stimulus.

THE ALL-OR-NONE LAW

The size of a neural response and the velocity of its conduction along the entire length of an axon are both independent of the magnitude of a stimulus. This all-or-none relationship states that once a stimulus is intense enough to initiate an impulse, the characteristics of that impulse will not be altered by any change in the properties of that stimulus.

This does not mean that changes in stimulus intensity do not have any effects on the conduction of nerve impulses. It means rather that information regarding stimulus intensity is coded in some way other than the size of the action potential or the speed of its conduction. The alternative involves time. The stronger the stimulus, the shorter the interval between the onset of the stimulus and the time for the action potential to reach its maximum amplitude. As a corollary, this also means that the stronger the stimulus, the greater the number of impulses that will be propagated per unit time up to a certain maximum. The reason for this limitation will become evident from a consideration of Fig. 1.7, which depicts the changes that occur in the resting potential during an action potential.

Inspection of the figure shows that following the depolarization of the neuron, the resting potential does not return immediately to its prestimulation level, but actually increases slightly below that level for a brief moment. This increased negativity is referred to as a hyperpolarization since the membrane is now more negatively polarized than before. This brief hyperpolarization condition has important implications for further nerve propagation since during this period, the intensity of the stimulus required to initiate an action potential must be increased to overcome the increased resting membrane potential. Actually, this hyperpolarization phase has two components, one an absolute refractory stage during which no stimulus, no matter how intense, is capable of initiating an action potential, and the other a relative refractory stage, during which only a superthreshold stimulus has any such effect.

The practical importance of this phenomenon is that the duration of the refractory period determines the maximum frequency with which a nerve fiber can transmit impulses. Inspection of Fig. 1.8 illustrates this principle by showing that the propagation of a second action potential can occur only if there is a certain minimum in the time between consecutive stimuli.

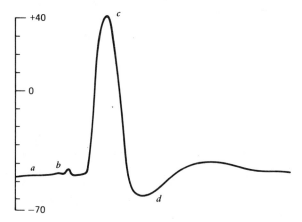

Fig. 1.7 Schematic diagram of an action potential. Vertical scale indicates the potential (mV) of the internal electrode relative to the external ionic concentration: (a) the resting membrane potential; (b) onset of stimulation; (c) maximum depolarization; (d) refractory period.

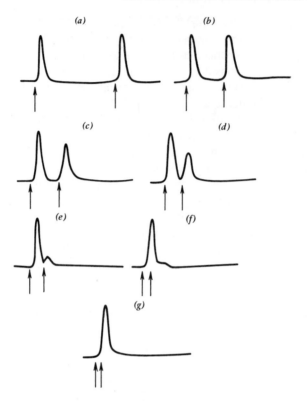

Fig. 1.8 Illustration of refractory period in the propagation of two action potentials. Arrows indicate excitatory impulses. Amplitudes are shown for various times following an initial stimulus. When the time between successive stimuli is relatively long (*a*), the amplitude of each action potential is the same. However, as the time interval is decreased, the amplitude of the second action potential decreases as the second stimulus enters the relative refractory period of the first (*b* to *f*). When the second stimulus falls into the absolute refractory period of the first (*g*), no impulse is generated by the second stimulus.

The fact that a very strong stimulus is capable of exciting a fiber during its relative refractory period offers yet another way in which the nervous system is able to differentiate between stimuli of different intensities. Since a strong stimulus can excite a nerve while it is in its relative refractory phase, the threshold does not have to return to its usual level for that stimulus to initiate a response. Hence the stronger the stimulus, the greater the impulse frequency.

Once neurophysiologists realized that the nervous system recognizes differences in stimulus intensity by means of changes in the frequency of neuronal discharge, the question then arose as to how great the increase in stimulus intensity had to be before it could be perceived. Thus if a room were lighted by 100 candles and another lighted candle were brought into the room, could the increase in brightness be detected?

The question, or at least one like it, was actually posed more than a century ago and its solution is stated in the psychophysical law proposed by Gustav Fechner (1801–1887): increments in the perceived intensity of a stimulus bear a logarithmic relation to the physical intensity of that stimulus. However, it was not until the development of modern electrophysiological techniques that this relationship between changes in the frequency of neuronal discharge (the neurophysiological correlate of sensation) and the logarithm of stimulus intensity were demonstrated experimentally (e.g., Matthews, 1931).

Nerve fibers, however, are not single neurons but rather collections of individual nerve cells. Therefore it should be kept in mind that each individual neuron in a nerve fiber has its own threshold, amplitude, and velocity of conduction, and should the electrical activity of the whole nerve be recorded, not one but several neurons would be fired. Such a record is referred to as the compound action potential of the nerve, since it is made up of the action potentials of several nerve cells.

The most convenient way of initiating an action potential in a nerve is by means of electric shocks because the parameters associated with this kind of stimulation may be controlled precisely and specified. Another advantage of using electrical shock stimulation is that it resembles the impulse generated in the nerve fiber. However, alterations in the resting membrane potential of a nerve cell may be brought about by almost any kind of stimulus change, provided it is sufficiently intense, quick, and localized. For example, pressure that is suddenly applied directly to a nerve induces an action potential. A sudden intense change in temperature similarly may give rise to an action potential.

This ability to excite nerve fibers by a variety of different stimuli can be appreciated by means of a simple experiment. If you close your eyes and then press on one of them in the area near the nose, a circle will be perceived on the side opposite to that being pressed. This demonstrates that it is possible to "see" even when there is no visual input.

The basis for this phenomenon hearkens back to the doctrine of the "specific energy of nerves" first proposed over a century ago by the German physiologist, Johannes Müller. In its simplest terms, this doctrine states that each of the sensory systems carries impulses from sensory receptors to specific areas of the brain, and sensory experience depends upon which area of the brain receives the stimulus input. In other words, the interpretation of sensory experience depends upon the area of the brain that receives the sensory impulse, no matter where or how that stimulation originates. Thus stimulation of any point in the visual system, for example, the retina, optic nerve, lateral geniculate, or visual cortex, will produce a visual sensation.

This phenomenon has important implications for the activity of certain drugs since it may be possible that the visual, auditory, tactile, and other hallucinations produced by drugs such as LSD result from their activity at certain sensory areas of the brain. For example, Oster (1970) has described a series of experiments involving electrical stimulation of the visual cortex in humans. Such stimulation causes the subject to perceive specks of light or vivid formlike patterns, depending upon the actual locus of the visual cortex being stimulated. Should certain drugs be able to mimic the effects of electrical stimulation in these same areas, it is possible that this aspect of their activity could account for many of the sensory effects associated with their use.

INTERNEURONAL COMMUNICATION: THE SYNAPSE

Up to this point, the discussion of the mechanism of the nerve impulse has been restricted to the individual nerve cell, with no consideration given to the passage of the impulse from one nerve cell to another. However, even in the simplest stimulus-response reflex arc, impulses are passed through either two or three nerve cells before any response is forthcoming. In fact, it is because nerve impulses are channeled through networks of nerve cells that complexity in behavior is possible.

Nerve cells are able to influence the activity of other nerve cells by one of two processes—synaptic or ephatic transmission. Synaptic transmission involves the passage of impulses from the synaptic terminals of axons to receptor areas in the dendrites or cell bodies of other nerve or muscle cells. Ephatic transmission, on the other hand, involves the transfer of impulses from axon to axon and occurs where axons are in such close proximity that the impulse in one neuron excites or inhibits an impulse in the nerve fibers adjacent to it. From a pharmacological standpoint, however, only the former means of neuronal communication is of interest since only synaptic transmission is mediated by chemical agents. Therefore, in the following discussion, no further attention is devoted to the process of ephatic transmission.

The first convincing evidence that interneuronal communication was chemically mediated was reported by Loewi in 1921. In a now classic experiment, Loewi first stimulated the vagus nerve of a perfused frog heart and then brought the perfusate into contact with a second frog heart. Stimulation of the vagus nerve quickly slowed the beat of the first heart, and shortly afterward the beat of the second heart was also slowed. Since there was no physical contact between the two hearts except via the perfusate, it was clear that whatever it was that had mediated this effect, it had to have been chemical in nature. Loewi called the substance released from the vagus nerve, "vagusstoff." Shortly thereafter he conducted a similar experiment, this time stimulating the nervus accelerans. This had the effect of increasing the beat of both hearts. Accordingly, he termed the chemical released from the accelerans nerve, "accleranstoff." These chemicals were subsequently identified as acetylcholine and norepinephrine, respectively. In 1934, Dale referred to the nerve fibers which release acetylcholine as "cholinergic" and those which release norepinephrine as "adrenergic" and these terms are still used to characterize nerve pathways that are mediated by these chemicals.

One of the most distinctive features of the presynaptic terminal boutons from which the neurotransmitters are released are the small vesiclelike structures located close to the terminal membrane (see Fig. 1.9). It is believed that these vesicles actually contain the chemicals that mediate the transmission of impulses across the synapse. However, in addition to this vesicular store of transmitter which is referred to as the "stable bound" or simply "bound" pool, there is a substantial amount of transmitter located in the cytoplasm of the axon terminal which is referred to as the "labile" or "free pool." The observation of small fluctuations in the resting potential of postsynaptic fibers (cf. Fatt and Katz, 1950) suggests that minute amounts of this labile pool of transmitter are constantly being released from presynaptic terminals, and this may account for the continuous electrical activity of the CNS. The transmitter stores located in the vesicles would thus represent a reserve transmitter pool (cf. Sotelo, 1971). It is the release of this reserve "bound" pool that often initiates an action potential in postsynaptic neurons.

The manner in which a depolarization entering the synaptic bouton causes the release of the transmitter, however, is still a matter of speculation, although it appears that Ca^{2+} ions are involved in the mechanism. This is suggested by the sharp rise in the influx of Ca^{2+} into the axoplasm of nerve fibers immediately prior to synaptic discharge (Hodgkins and Keyes, 1957) and by the decrease in the amount of transmitter that is released when the concentration of Ca^{2+} ions in the extracellular fluid is reduced (del Castello and Katz, 1954).

Apparently, upon entering the synaptic bouton, a depolarizing current induces an influx of Ca^{2+} ions, which causes the vesicles in the bouton to move toward and to fuse with the cell membrane. This fusion then results in the discharge of neurotransmitter. This view of the synaptic discharge is referred to as the exocytosis vesicular hypothesis. Interestingly, prolonged electrical stimulation of nerve fibers has been found to either increase or

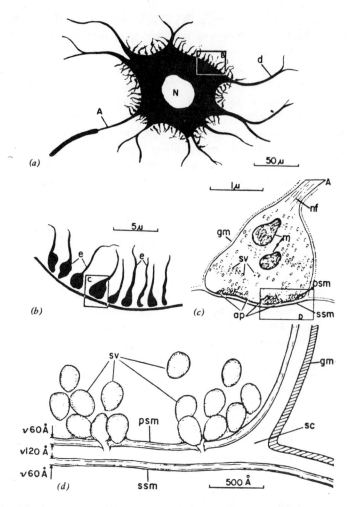

Fig. 1.9 Diagram showing boutonlike synaptic junctions at different magnifications with the optical and electron microscope. (*a*) The nucleus (N), the axon (A), and the dendrites (d) are indicated. Numerous boutonlike endings make synaptic contact with the surface of the perikaryon (axosomatic junctions) and of the dendrites (axodendritic junctions). Enclosure B is magnified five times in (*b*). (*b*) End feet (e), as seen under high magnification with the optical microscope. The afferent axons are enlarged at the endings. The presence of mitochondria is indicated. Enclosure C is magnified about six times with the electron microscope. (*c*) Mitochondria (m), neuroprotofibrils (nf), and synaptic vesicles (sv) are shown within the ending. Three clusters of synaptic vesicles become attached to the presynaptic membrane (psm); these are probably active points (ap) of the synapse. Both the presynaptic psm and the subsynaptic membrane (ssm) show higher electron density. The glial membrane is shown in dotted lines (gm). Enclosure D is magnified about 10 times in (*d*). (*d*) Diagram of the synaptic membrane as observed with high-resolution electron microscopy (see text). Some synaptic vesicles (sv) are seen attached to the psm and opening into the synaptic cleft (sc) (from De Robertis, 1959).

decrease the number of synaptic vesicles depending upon the frequency with which the nerve is stimulated (DeRobertis and Vas Ferreira, 1957).

An increase in the efficiency of synaptic transmission has in fact been proposed by several theorists as the neurophysiological change underlying the phenomenon of learning (for example, Hebb, 1949; Young, 1951; Eccles, 1953; Kandel and Spencer, 1969). These formulations are derived from Lashley's (1950) hypothesis that learning involves the formation of an "engram," a spatiotemporal sequence of neuronal events occurring in the brain. With continued activation of the engram subserving a particular learned response, it is proposed that the synapses in the neuronal circuit of the engram become more efficient with the result that impulses are passed through the circuit with increasing facility each time a certain stimulus complex is encountered.

NEUROTRANSMITTERS: CRITERIA FOR THEIR IDENTIFICATION

Although there is no longer any doubt that communication between neurons in the mammalian nervous system is mediated by chemical substances that are released from terminal boutons, the identity of these neurotransmitters is still unknown for the most part. Although acetylcholine and norepinephrine have long been recognized as transmitters in the parasympathetic and sympathetic divisions of the autonomic nervous system, it is only relatively recently that these chemicals have been shown to be present in the brain. However, because of their activity at peripheral synapses and their presence in the CNS, substances such as acetylcholine and norepinephrine are obvious candidates for the role of transmitters in the CNS as well. If this is the case and if it can be shown that these chemicals are involved in behaviors such as eating, drinking, sleep, and sex, then it may be possible to affect these behaviors by administering drugs which are able to mimic, enhance, or interfere with their activity. However, for a chemical to be an actual neurotransmitter, not only must its presence be demonstrated, but also it must satisfy a number of additional criteria. Most of these criteria are derived from facts that are known concerning the mechanisms of release, action, and inactivation of acetylcholine in the peripheral nervous system (Curtis, 1961).

The requirements that must be satisfied before a substance can be accepted even as a potential candidate for synaptic transmission are as follows.

1. It must be present in the area of the synapse. This is obvious. But to mediate neural transmission, the transmitter must not only be present in the vicinity of its site of action, but also be available at exactly the moment it is needed. This means that the enzymes that synthesize the transmitter

should also be present in the vicinity of the synapse. The absence of such enzymes, however, does not completely invalidate a substance as a neurotransmitter, since some of the transmitter could be taken back up by the bouton from which it was liberated, and the remainder could be synthesized in the soma and then passed along to the bouton by a process of axoplasmic transport.

2. When released, the transmitter must be detectable in the extracellular fluid in the vicinity of the synapse. With modern collection methods and techniques such as the push-pull cannula and cerebroventricular perfusion, it has been shown in the case of acetylcholine that not only is this substance released into the synapse, but that the extent of its release is roughly proportional to the electrical activity going on in a particular area of the brain (Mitchell, 1963).

3. After being released from presynaptic terminals, the neurotransmitter must act upon its receptors in the postsynaptic membrane. With the aid of specialized techniques, it is possible to apply small amounts of putative neurontransmitters to the same areas as those that are activated by endogenously occurring chemicals. A similarity in effects between the actions of exogenous and endogenous substances provides impressive evidence for the molecular identity of the naturally occurring transmitter (Werman, 1966).

4. A mechanisms for terminating the activity of the transmitter must be present in the vicinity of the synapse. If the transmitter were not inactivated, it might produce a relatively long-lasting depolarization or hyperpolarization which could prevent further neuronal transmission in the postsynaptic nerve cell. This inactivating mechanism might involve an enzyme that degrades the transmitter, a reuptake of the transmitter by presynaptic terminals, or a diffusion of the transmitter away from the receptor and into the bloodstream. From there it could be transported to an active site of destruction remote from the area of the receptor.

An alternative means of terminating the activity of a transmitter could be through the actions of a second transmitter whose effects are opposite to the first. This suggests the possibility of a recurrent collateral pathway—a neuron in an excited state stimulates an adjacent neuron, causing it to liberate a transmitter which acts to inhibit the first cell. By means of a contiguous anatomical relationship between cells, a negative feedback loop would terminate the activity induced by a neuron in less than 2 msec (Anderson et al., 1964a). Such circuits have actually been located in several areas of the central nervous system (Anderson et al., 1964a, 1964b) and are reminiscent of Hebb's cell assembly hypothesis which he implicates in the phenomena of learning and perception (Hebb, 1949).

5. If in addition to satisfying all these criteria, a particular substance were found to resemble the transmitter in terms of its pharmacological activity, the evidence for the identity of that substance with the naturally occurring transmitter would be quite compelling (Curtis, 1961).

At present, no specific chemical substance is able to fulfill all these criteria. Some of those that have been considered, however, are acetylcholine, norepinephrine, dopamine, 5-hydroxytryptamine, histamine, glutamine, Gaba, and substance P, but only the first four have been investigated in any detail. Consequently the latter four are not considered further.

ACETYLCHOLINE

Acetylcholine, its precursors, and the enzymes responsible for its synthesis and inactivation have all been located in various areas of the brain.

The principal reaction involved in the formation of acetylcholine (ACh) is the acetylation of choline by acetyl coenzyme A. This reaction is catalyzed by the enzyme choline acetyltransferase (also called choline acetylase). The distribution of choline acetyltransferase in the CNS has been described by various investigators. Although its activity varies with the extent of cortical maturation (Hebb and Silver, 1956), its distribution is roughly parallel to that of ACh (see Table 1.2), the highest concentrations being found in the motor cortex with little or no activity occurring in the cerebellum. Although little activity is found in the optic nerve, it is interesting to note that a substantial amount of these substances occurs in the retina and the lateral geniculate body (Hebb and Silver, 1956).

The "rate-limiting factor" in the formation of ACh is believed to be choline since interference with its availability markedly reduces endogenous levels of ACh in nerve tissue. During synaptic transmission, choline is reabsorbed back into the neuron following the reaction of ACh and its receptors and its subsequent hydrolysis into choline and acetate. However, the source of the substances that combine to produce choline originally is unknown at present. The synthesis and inactivation of ACh are summarized in Fig. 1.10.

Evidence that choline is the "rate-limiting factor" in the synthesis of ACh has been shown by several investigators (e.g., MacIntosh et al., 1956, 1958; Gardiner, 1961) using hemicholinium (HC-3), a compound which has certain structural resemblances to choline. Apparently, this substance blocks the uptake of choline into the cell by successfully competing for the carriers that normally transport extracellular choline to the intracellular sites at which it is acetylated to ACh (MacIntosh, 1959). As a result, it ultimately prevents synaptic transmission in cholinergic fibers by depleting ACh stores. However, hemicholinium does not cross the blood-brain barrier readily and therefore its effects are confined mainly to the peripheral nervous system, thus limiting its use as a tool for studying central mechanisms believed to be cholinergically mediated. On the other hand, should the drug be placed directly into the CNS, a rapid decrease in whole brain levels of ACh would ensue (cf. Gardiner, 1961).

Once ACh has reacted with its receptors, its activity must be terminated so that the postsynaptic membrane can repolarize and be ready to respond once more. The enzyme that inactivates ACh is cholinesterase. Actually

Table 1.2   Acetylcholine and Choline Acetyltransferase in the Central Nervous System of the Cat[a]

Tissue	Acetylcholine Content[b]	Choline Acetyltransferase Content[b]
Medulla	1–2.7	—
Pons	1.4–5.0	—
Thalamus	1.5–4.5	1.7–3.5
Hypothalamus	1.6–2.1	—
Cerebellar cortex	0.1–0.3	0.01–0.2
Olfactory bulb	1.3	0.79–2.2
Superior colliculus	4.5	2.0–5.4
Optic nerve	0	0

[a] Values taken from Hebb, 1957; Feldberg, 1945; and Phillis, 1970.
[b] Values are expressed as $\mu g/g$ fresh tissue.

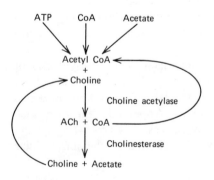

Fig. 1.10   Biosynthesis of acetylcholine.

two types of cholinesterase exist at different sites, one specific for ACh and the other nonspecific. The first is called either acetylcholinesterase (AChE), true or specific cholinesterase, or cholinesterase I (ChE I). The second is called pseudo or nonspecific cholinesterase, butyrocholinesterase (BuChE), or cholinesterase II (ChE II). In general, ACh is found in neural tissue whereas BuChE is located in nonneural tissue, especially plasma. This accounts for the rapid inactivation of ACh when it is administered parenterally. However, almost all the pharmacological effects of the anticholinesterase agents are due to inhibition of AchE rather than inhibition of BuChE. Moreover, the distribution of AChE closely parallels that of ACh, so much so that the presence of AChE is often taken as indicative of ACh's presence (Friede, 1966).

The total amount of ACh in the brain bears a direct inverse relationship to CNS activity. For instance, during anesthesia, when the electrical activity of the brain is reduced, the content of ACh in the brain increases; on the other hand, direct electrical stimulation of the brain, or the convulsant action of certain drugs, tends to decrease brain levels of ACh (Richter and Crossland, 1949; Elliot et al., 1950; Tobias et al., 1946). Mitchell (1963), in fact, has demonstrated that ACh is released from synaptic terminals and that this release bears a close relationship to the electrical activity in the brain. Thus these data also support another of the criteria recommending ACh for the role of central neurotransmitter. Despite its rapid synthesis, however, the amount of ACh in nerve terminals tends to remain at a fairly constant level (MacIntosh, 1963). Apparently the synthesis of ACh continues even when the vesicles binding it become saturated. Any excess ACh presumably is inactivated by minute amounts of AChE located in presynaptic terminals (MacIntosh, 1963).

After its release from synaptic vesicles, ACh diffuses across the synaptic cleft and it is believed that it reacts with a specific receptor located on the postsynaptic cell membrane. The evidence for the existence of specialized chemical receptors is mainly inferential and is discussed at length in a later chapter. For the moment, a receptor will be defined as "a genetically-determined tissue component which has been designed to interact with a naturally occurring substance, this interaction initiating a series of events culminating in an effect" (Ehrenpreis et al., 1970).

At some receptors in the peripheral nervous system, for example, those in the heart and smooth muscle, ACh produces an effect quite similar to that of muscarine, a poison found in certain species of mushroom, and for historical reasons, these effects of ACh are termed muscarinic. In character, muscarinic effects are similar to those occurring as a result of stimulation in the parasympathetic nervous system, for example, slowing of the heart, constriction of the pupils of the eye, and relaxation of the sphincters of the stomach. At other receptors, for example, sympathetic ganglia and skeletal neuromuscular junctions, ACh acts as nicotine does, producing first an excitation caused by a depolarization of the postsynaptic membrane, and then depression caused by persistent depolarization. Such effects are appropriately termed nicotinic. Using microiontophoretic techniques which permit the application of ACh directly into discrete areas of tissue, the cholinergic receptors of the brain have been found to be primarily muscarinic in activity.

Although several investigators have shown that ACh produces excitation in the CNS (e.g., Krnjevic and Phillis, 1963; Spehlmann, 1965), certain observations connected with these effects have raised some doubts concerning the actual role of ACh in the brain. For instance, the onset of the response to exogenously administered ACh in the brain is quite slow compared to its relatively rapid onset when applied to Renshaw cells (Krnjevic et al., 1971). Acetylcholine has been found additionally to depolarize not only neurons, but also glia cells which act as supportive tissue for neural cells. Finally, the fact that ACh depolarizes nerve cells in the brain without altering their membrane resistance (Krnjevic and Schintz, 1967) likewise does not agree well with the sequence of events typically occurring during synaptic transmission in the peripheral nervous system. It is possible, however, that the mechanisms responsible for the initiation of an action potential in the CNS are in some way different from those in the peripheral nervous system, and therefore these anomalies do not invalidate ACh as a neural transmitter.

There is also the possibility that in some areas of the brain, ACh may initiate a neural response indirectly by causing the release of other substances such as norepinephrine, which then acts on postsynaptic fibers to initiate an action potential. This, in essence, is the Burn-Rand (1962) hypothesis. The evidence for this proposal comes from experiments showing that the removal of norepinephrine from neuronal stores by either degeneration of sympathetic nerves or by reserpine (see p. 160) causes ACh and nicotine to be ineffective in eliciting a response in autonomic effector cells although this had been possible before the depletion of norepinephrine. Consequently, some hypothesis like that proposed by Burn and Rand may account ultimately for certain of the anomalies surrounding ACh's activity in the brain.

What is perhaps even more challenging to any attempt to assess the role of ACh as a transmitter in the CNS is the observation that this substance appears to have excitatory effects at some neurons in the brain and depressant effects at others. For example, out of a total population of 600 neurons in the pons and medulla, 35.5% were excited by iontophoretic applications of ACh, whereas 22% were inhibited. The remaining 42.5% were unresponsive (Bradley et al., 1966). Excitatory and inhibitory effects associated with ACh also have been observed in the hypothalamus (Bloom et al., 1963). Results, such as these suggest that there are possibly two distinct receptors for ACh, one excitatory, the other inhibitory. This singularly points out the folly of designating ACh an excitatory transmitter. As pointed out by Bradley (1968), the reason ACh may have been so regarded in the past is that only excitatory effects were observed at neuromuscular junctions following application of ACh. On the basis of its effects at the peripheral nervous system, investigators merely assumed a similar action centrally. This generalization obviously must be reconsidered.

It appears then that in many instances, ACh does not fulfill the physiological criterion of "identity of action" (cf. Werman, 1963). In addition, there are also pharmacological data that raise some difficulties concerning its putative transmitter function in the CNS. For instance, in very low concentrations, exogenously applied ACh produces capillary dilation in the rabbit ear. Although the cholinergic blocking agent atropine is able to antagonize this pharmacological effect, when the dilation is produced by the stimulation of the pertinent sensory fibers in this area, atropine no longer has this blocking effect (Halton and Perry, 1951). Similar findings have been reported by Ritchie and Armett (1963). This means that although ACh is able to mimic the effects of the naturally occurring transmitter (whose actions induce dilation), ACh itself may not be that physiological transmitter.

Despite all these anomalies connected wtih its activity, however, the evidence linking ACh with the transmission of impulses at some synapses in the CNS is impressive and the role of ACh as a neurotransmitter in the brain is, therefore, not implausible.

CATECHOLAMINES: NOREPINEPHRINE AND DOPAMINE

The presence of both norepinephrine and epinephrine in the mammalian brain was reported as early as 1946 by von Euler, but at that time no distinction was made between them. Instead, they were referred to as a single substance called "sympathin." Four years later, Holtz (1950) corroborated von Euler's observations and demonstrated that nearly all the "sympathin" in the CNS was actually norepinephrine. In 1954, Vogt initiated what is still an active research program in this area, namely, the functional role of the catecholamines in the CNS. As part of her attempt to ascertain the answer to this question, she described in detail the distribution of norepinephrine in the dog and cat brain, and shortly thereafter hypotheses began appearing relating the possible interplay between these amines and the behavioral effects of drugs (cf. Brodie et al., 1959). Also at this time, the presence of a third catecholamine, dopamine, was detected in the mammalian brain (Weil-Malherbe and Bone, 1957) and hypotheses were soon being directed at its role as well.

In this section, the evidence linking the catecholamines in the mediation of synaptic transmission is reviewed. The behavioral effects of drugs that cause the release or enhancement of these catecholamines are discussed in a later chapter.

The formation of the catecholamines in brain tissue begins with the conversion of the naturally occurring amino acid tyrosine to dopa by the enzyme tyrosine hydroxylase, in the presence of oxygen. Tyrosine hydroxylase is ubiquitous in the brain (Nagatsu et al., 1964) but is found in relatively small amounts and is therefore the "rate-limiting factor" in the production of the catecholamines. Analogues of tyrosine such as α-methyl-p-tyrosine which inhibit the activity of tyrosine hydroxylase are able to reduce the catecholamine content of the brain to a much greater extent than is possible with drugs that inhibit the activity of other enzymes that take part in the biosynthesis of these substances (see below).

Once dopa is formed from tyrosine, it is converted into dopamine by the enzyme dopa decarboxylase. The highest concentrations of dopa decarboxylase are found in the caudate nucleus. Lower amounts are found in the hypothalamus, brain stem, reticular formation, septal region, and olfactory tubercle. The least amounts occur in the cerebral neocortex and cerebellum (Kuntzman et al., 1961; Bertler and Rosengren, 1959). The activity of this enzyme can also be inhibited, but the effect on the catecholamine content of the brain is relatively minimal compared to that following administration of α-methyl-p-tyrosine.

The third step involves the conversion of dopamine to norepinphrine in the presence of oxygen by the copper-containing enzyme dopamine-β-oxidase. Dopamine-β-oxidase is located in those areas of the brain in which catecholamine metabolism is quite high. The greatest concentrations are thus to be found in the hypothalamus; the lowest concentrations are found in the cerebellum and the cerebral cortex (Udenfriend and Creveling, 1959). Inhibition of this enzyme by agents such as disulfiram tends to reduce the levels of norepinephrine, but increases those of dopamine in the brain.

Dopamine itself appears to play a double role in brain tissue. On the one hand, it acts as a precursor for norepinephrine, and the concentration of dopamine in some areas of the brain is thus roughly proportional to that of norepinephrine (Kuntzman et al., 1961). However, dopamine is also found in rather high concentrations in the caudate nucleus where norepinephrine levels are quite low. This suggests that dopamine may be involved as a synaptic transmitter in the caudate nucleus and possibly in other areas of the brain as well (Hornkiewicz, 1966). A detailed description of the relative distribution of dopamine and norepinephrine in the mammalian brain is presented in Table 1.3.

Table 1.3   Concentration of Norepinephrine and Dopamine in the Central Nervous System of the Cat[a]

Tissue	Norepinephrine Content[b]	Dopamine Content[b]
Medulla	0.39	0.08
Pons	0.20–0.52	0.11
Cerebellum	0.13	0.02
Thalamus	0.22	0.05–0.50
Hypothalamus	2.05	0.75
Basal ganglia	0.22	8.00
Cerebral cortex	0.28	0.07

[a] Values are from Phillis, 1970.

[b] Values are expressed as $\mu g/g$ fresh tissue.

Although dopamine may play some part of its own in synaptic transmission, it is now generally agreed that norepinephrine is the principal catecholamine in the CNS. Table 1.3 shows that the highest concentrations of this amine are located in the hypothalamus; the lowest concentrations occur in the cerebellum and olfactory bulb. Despite the fact that the turnover rate of norepinephrine in the CNS is fairly rapid (cf. Spector et al., 1962), brain norepinephrine levels appear to be fairly stable over a period of time regardless of neuronal activity. Apparently, this is because the rate of conversion of tyrosine to dopa is affected by the levels of norepinephrine in a kind of negative feedback mechanism (Cooper et al., 1970).

The final step in the synthesis of the catecholamines is the conversion of norepinephrine into epinephrine by the enzyme phenylethanolamine-N-methyltransferase. Howevr, though there is a relatively high concentration of epinephrine in the brain of the chicken, only a very small amount of this catecholamine can be detected in the mammalian CNS and its function there has yet to be determined.

The various steps in the biosynthesis of epinephrine from tyrosine are summarized in Fig. 1.11. Once norepinephrine has been released from its terminals, there is no enzyme resembling acetycholinesterase to cause its total destruction. Instead, inactivation occurs by means of a number of processes, the least of which involves enzymatic activity. Most of the physiological activity of norepinephrine is terminated by its reabsorption into

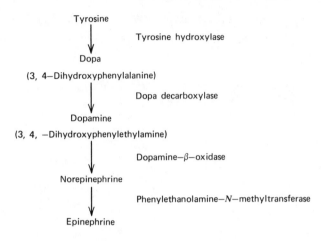

Fig. 1.11   Biosynthesis of the catecholamines.

adrenergic nerves. Some of this norepinephrine is taken into synaptic vesicles for reuse. The rest is inactivated by the enzyme monoamine oxidase (MAO), which is located in the mitochondria of the bouton. Norepinephrine that is not taken back into adrenergic nerves flows into the circulation and is metabolized by the enzyme catechol-*o*-methyltransferase (COMT). The actual importance of these two enzymatic steps in the inactivation of norepinephrine is indicated by the fact that even with the total inhibition of COMT and MAO, the effect of exogenously administered norepinephrine is still terminated rapidly (Crout, 1961). An estimate of the percentage of infused norepinephrine removed by the various mechanisms available for its inactivation is presented in Table 1.4.

In light of the rapid uptake of norepinephrine back into nerve cells, evidence for the release of this substance following stimulation of nerve fibers has been negligible (cf. McLennan, 1970); therefore, its detectability following release from its synapses cannot be used to evaluate norepinephrine's role as a physiological transmitter.

Table 1.4   Fate of Infused Norepinephrine[a]

Absorption by adrenergic nerve fibers	60%
Inactivation by COMT	15%
Inactivation in liver	20%
Interaction with receptors	5%

[a] From Bhagat (1971).

Little is known regarding the actual mechanism by which the release of norepinephrine occurs except that Ca^{2+} ions again appear to be involved in the process. Once it is released from its synaptic storage sites, norepinephrine diffuses across the synaptic cleft and reacts with a specific receptor located on the postsynaptic cell membrane. This results either in a depolarization or a hyperpolarization of the postsynaptic neuron. On the basis of pharmacological evidence, there appear to be two basic types of adrenergic receptors which can be differentiated according to their responsiveness to various sympathomimetic amines and according to their differential susceptibility to blockade by drugs.

These two types of receptors have been designated as α and β by Ahlquist (1948). The α receptors are differentially more responsive to norepinephrine than epinephrine or isoproterenol and are selectively blocked by drugs such as phenoxybenzamine. At the β receptors, the order of activity is reversed, with isoproterenol being most active and norepinephrine being less so. These β receptors can be blocked by drugs such as propranolol. It should be pointed out, however, that this separation of adrenergic receptors has been based on studies of drugs acting at the peripheral nervous system and therefore may not be totally applicable to the type of adrenergic receptor found in the CNS.

The various experiments dealing with the problem of "transmitter identity" of the adrenergic neural chemical have been summarized by McLennan (1971, pp. 114–115, Table 2). In general, the most predominant effect is that of depression of neuronal activity. However, since no comparisons have been made between the effects of norepinephrine and those of stimulation of adrenergic fibers, it is difficult to judge whether these effects are due to a true inhibitory effect of norepinephrine or a general nonspecific depression (McLennan, 1971).

Studies of the pharmacological resemblance between dopamine and norepinephrine and the transmitter at certain synapses, however, have proved more encouraging. For example, the adrenergic blocking compound phenoxybenzamine has been shown to prevent the depressant effects of dopamine and those of electrical stimulation at the same neuron in the caudate nucleus (York, 1967; York and McLennan, 1967). Similarly, the blocking agent dibenamine has been found to depress synaptic activity in olfactory bulb neurons produced by both norepinephrine and direct stimulation of olfactory fibers (Bloom et al., 1964). On the other hand, there are also data showing the pharmacological blockade of effects produced by norepinephrine but not by those produced by direct stimulation of neural fibers (Yamamoto, 1967).

In summary, the data supporting norepinephrine's and dopamine's roles as transmitters are not nearly as impressive as those involving acetylcholine.

However, on the basis of the distribution of these substances and their precursors, the evidence is still encouraging and their candidacy still cannot be dismissed (cf. McLennan, 1971).

SEROTONIN

5-hydroxytryptamine (5-HT), which is also known as serotonin, is found throughout the CNS (see Table 1.5). However, there is even less information bearing on its candidacy as a synaptic transmitter than there is involving norepinephrine. Nevertheless, because it is distributed so widely in the brain and because the distribution of its precursors roughly parallels its own distribution, there is a strong probability that serotonin is also involved in synaptic transmission in some areas of the brain.

Table 1.5 Distribution of Serotonin in the Central Nervous System of the Dog[a]

Tissue	Serotonin Content[b]
Medulla	0.62
Pons	0.38
Cerebellum	0.0.09
Thalamus	0.57
Hypothalamus	0.64
Cerebral cortex	0.17

[a] From Bogdanski et al. (1957).
[b] Values are expressed as $\mu g/g$ fresh tissue.

The first step in the formation of this amine involves the conversion of dietary tryptophan to 5-hydroxytryptophan (5-HTP) by the enzyme tryptophan hydroxylase. Tryptophan hydroxylase is the rate-limiting enzyme in the formation of serotonin and has its highest activity in the hypothalamus and thalamus; least activity is found in the cerebellum and cerebral cortex (Grahame-Smith, 1964a, 1964b). Most of this enzyme is located in the mitochondrial fraction of the nerve cell.

The next step involves the conversion of 5-HTP to 5-hydroxytryptamine, a reaction that is catalyzed by the enzyme 1-amino acid decarboxylase. This enzyme, also called dopa decarboxylase or 5-HTP decarboxylase, is the same enzyme as that which converts dopa to dopamine. The regional distribution of 1-amino acid decarboxylase nearly parallels that of

5-HT in the entire brain except for the limbic system (Udenfriend et al., 1957). The steps in the synthesis of serotonin are summarized in Fig. 1.12.

The inactivation of 5-HT is somewhat similar to that of norepinephrine, since for the most part 5-HT is broken down by monoamine oxidase (to 5-hydroxyindole acetic acid, 5HIAA). The distribution of MAO in relation to 5-HT has been described by Bogdanski et al. (1957).

No information is available at this time concerning the release of 5-HT during stimulation of nerve tissues (McLennan, 1970). However, a summary of the literature dealing with the application of 5-HT to isolated neurons can be found in McLennan (1970, pp. 114–115, Table 2). Of all the neurons in the pons and medulla tested by Bradley (1968), as many as 90% responded to the application of 5-HT, half with excitation, the other half with inhibition. In this regard, Roberts and Straughan (1957) have presented data suggesting that there may be in fact two specific receptors for 5-HT, since only the excitatory effects of this amine are antagonized by LSD-25; the inhibitory effects are not.

EXCITATION AND INHIBITION

After a neurotransmitter has been released from its presynaptic terminals, it diffuses across the synapse and in some way or another causes a change in the ionic permeability of the postsynaptic membrane. This results in a nonpropagated local response in the postsynaptic resting membrane potential. Two different kinds of local responses may be generated. One involves a depolarization of the membrane potential such that it becomes less negative. This depolarization is produced when the membrane's permeability to sodium ions is increased and is known as an excitatory postsynaptic potential (EPSP). The other involves a hyperpolarization of the membrane potential such that the interior of the cell becomes more negative. This is called an inhibitory postsynaptic potential (IPSP) and is thought to occur as a result of either the outward flow of potassium ions or the inward flow of negatively charged chloride ions, or a combination

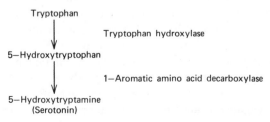

Fig. 1.12 Biosynthesis of serotonin.

of both. Although these local responses are in some ways similar to action potentials, it should be noted once more that these responses are not propagated but instead are confined to the membrane at which they are initiated. In addition, it is important to note that the nerve cell responds to the algebraic sum of the internal cell voltages. If the depolarization reaches the threshold level, an action potential will be triggered and a nerve impulse will be generated in the axon. The IPSP acts to reduce the probability of a near threshold stimulus producing an action potential.

Actually, there are two mechanisms of synaptic inhibition operating in the nervous system; one affects presynaptic, the other, postsynaptic activity.

In presynaptic inhibition, the terminal boutons synapse not on the dendrites or cell body of another cell but on the terminal boutons of other cells. This causes any depolarization in this area to be reduced, thus affecting the release of neurotransmitter. This type of inhibition is found in connection with the primary afferent pathways to the brain. By means of diminishing the activity in these pathways by such presynaptic inhibition, the internuncial neurons are thus able to suppress certain kinds of sensory input before they can activate the sensory areas of the brain (see p. 47). In effect, this mechanism may act as a perceptual gate (at the level of the spinal cord) screening out all sensory inputs which are of no importance to the organism (Eccles, 1963).

The principal form of inhibition taking place in the brain itself, however, is postsynaptic inhibition. In many of its characteristics, postsynaptic inhibition resembles postsynaptic excitation except for its resultant effect. This resemblance suggests that a nearly identical mechanism serves both. The main difference is that excitation involves a depolarization, whereas postsynaptic inhibition involves a hyperpolarization of the postsynaptic cell.

SUMMATION

The amount of neurotransmitter that is released from a single bouton is not great enough to depolarize a postsynaptic cell to the extent that an action potential will be triggered. However, if a number of boutons release their transmitter simultaneously, the algebraic sum of each of these individual amounts (quanta) of transmitter may be able to do so. As in the case of inhibition, so too with summation, there are two kinds possible. The first, called spatial summation, refers to the additive effects of transmitter substances that are released from several different presynaptic neurons. Together these quanta may sum up to produce a depolarization large enough to initiate an action potential, whereas none of these quanta would be individually capable of lowering the resting potential sufficiently enough to do so.

The second kind of summation is temporal. This refers to the additive effect of repeated discharges of transmitter from the same bouton. This can occur if stimulation of the presynaptic fiber is rapid enough so that there is some lingering effect of the first release of transmitter by the time that the second release arrives. However, since the probability of a neuron secreting enough transmitter on its own to depolarize a second neuron is not very great, spatial summation is a more realistic state of affairs than is temporal summation. Moreover, spatial summation is satisfied by the convergence of several synaptic terminals on a single receptor site. The possibility still exists, however, that spatial and temporal summation can occur simultaneously.

Summation thus refers to the ability of a neuron to react to stimuli which reach it at different times (temporal summation) or from different places (spatial summation) with a more intense response than would be the case if these stimuli were responded to individually. This phenomenon has a direct counterpart in behavior. For example, consider the actions of the blowfly when exposed to sugar solutions, as studied by Dethier (1953). The front legs of the blowfly contain very sensitive hairs which are used to detect food. When substances such as sugar solutions are encountered, the blowfly extends its proboscis and begins to feed. Dethier observed that if only one of the blowfly's legs were dipped into a sugar solution, the lowest concentration to which 50% of these animals would respond was 0.0037 M. On the other hand, if both legs were placed into the sugar solution, thus causing them both to be stimulated at the same time, summation would occur, as indicated by the fact that the lowest concentration to which 50% of the animals now responded was 0.0018 M.

Neurophysiological summation also has a counterpart in the activity of drugs. For instance, drugs for which a threshold exists in the dose-response function may have subthreshold effects that cannot be observed because the dose is too low. The effects of this same dose can be made observable, however, if the drug is given in conjunction with some other drug. For example, independent administration of drug A or B in subthreshold dosages may have effects that are not sufficiently intense enough to produce a measurable effect on their own. Given in combination, however, a small dose of B may be sufficient to increase the stimulus value of A so that it is now capable of eliciting an observable response.

When two drugs act to produce such an increased response, the phenomenon is termed "synergism." If the synergism is simply additive, it is referred to as summation. On the other hand, if two drugs acting in concert produce an effect greater than the sum of the two dosages given individually, this kind of synergism is referred to as potentiation.

CONVERGENCE AND DIVERGENCE

In the case of spatial summation, impulses traveling down axons of similar length and diameter may reach their synaptic boutons at about the same time. Therefore, the discharge of transmitter from each bouton may occur almost simultaneously. Such a pattern of synaptic events is termed convergence and represents the neuroanatomical basis for the phenomenon of summation.

Whereas convergence increases the probability that a stimulus will produce some response, divergent conduction decreases this possibility because it has the effect of dispersing impulses as more and more synapses are approached. This anatomical arrangement permits the screening out of irrelevant sensory information at progressive stages in the synaptic ladder so that ultimately, the organism is able to respond on a selective basis to stimuli that are relevant to its existence (Hebb, 1966). Divergent conduction is thus another of the ways the nervous system has for filtering the transmission of impulses to the brain.

THE SENSORY SYSTEM

In order to obtain information about its environment, an organism must possess an apparatus capable of (1) detecting stimulation, (2) transducing or coding that stimulation into electrical impulses, and (3) transmitting this information to specific areas of the nervous system including the brain for analysis. The way in which impulses are transmitted in the nervous system has already been discussed. In this section, the mechanisms that receive and transduce information are examined briefly.

The parts of the nervous system that have been especially modified to detect stimulation are the sensory receptors, of which there are four main types, the exteroceptor, the interoceptor, the proprioceptor, and the nociceptor. The exteroceptors respond to stimulation in the external environment such as light, sound, and smell; the interoceptors signal impulses arising from within the body such as the viscera; the proprioceptors are designed to detect input arising from the locomotor system of the body; and the nociceptors signal pain (see Table 1.6).

Although each receptor is specialized so as to signal different sensory events, each receptor basically responds to one of five different kinds of sensation. These are mechanical (deformation of cells, sound), temperature (hot and cold), pain, electromagnetic energy (light), and chemical (taste, odor). The type of sensation that is experienced when receptors are activated by one of these forms of energy is determined not by the stimulus

Table 1.6 General Classification of Sensory Receptors

Class	Sensation	Location
Exteroceptors	Sight, sound, smell, taste, cutaneous pain, cutaneous heat, cutaneous cold, cutaneous pressure	Body surfaces (detect stimuli outside the organism)
Interoceptors	Smell, taste, organic pain, organic heat, organic cold, organic pressure	Interior of body (detect stimuli originating from within the organism)
Proprioceptors	Movements in muscles, tendons, and joints; vestibular feedback (balance)	Muscles, tendons, joints, non-auditory parts of inner ear (detect movement)
Nociceptors	Cutaneous pain, organic pain, kinesthetic (movement-related) pain	Throughout body (detect noxious stimulation)

itself, but rather by the specific area of the brain in which the nerves carrying that energy terminate (law of specific nerve energies).

When a stimulus activates a particular sensory receptor, it causes a local flow of electrical current around the nerve endings of the receptor. This local current is produced as a result of a depolarization called a receptor or generator potential, which if great enough (i.e., suprathreshold) will initiate an action potential. Although the mechanism by which receptor potentials are generated varies with each particular receptor, in general receptor potentials occur as a result of an increased permeability of the receptor cell to certain ions such as sodium.

Once a receptor has been activated, it signals the intensity of a stimulus in one of two ways. The first we are already familiar with: the more intense the stimulus, the greater the frequency of discharge by the receptor. Alternatively, if the receptor adapts rather slowly, a strong stimulus will produce a greater number of impulses than a weak stimulus. In the case of adaptation, the frequency of discharge is high but it gradually falls off though the stimulus intensity remains the same. Another possibility is that a receptor simply becomes fatigued and is no longer able to discharge.

Although sensory receptors give rise to electrical impulses that are sent along sensory pathways, these impulses do not go directly to the brain. Instead, the information travels along a specific pathway which synapses along the way with specialized sensory nuclei called sensory relays. As a result of passing through these relays, the neural information arising from the receptors is often recoded. Additional recoding also takes place in the sensory areas of the brain to which the original sensory information was directed. Thus, in passing from receptor to brain, sensory information is subjected to various intermediate stages during which it is processed and further processed.

In addition, the nervous system also contains a special sensory feedback mechanism by which the CNS selects at the level of the sensory relays the kinds of information that will be passed on to the brain. This sensory feedback system is essentially a filtering mechanism by which information can be either rejected as being unimportant, or passed on for further analysis. This can be accomplished because of the pattern of excitatory and inhibitory neurons that impinge on the sensory relays. This causes them to become either depolarized or hyperpolarized, with the result that information coming into the relay will either produce an action potential in the neurons leading from the relay to the next station, or will not do so. On a behavioral level, this enables an organism to focus its attention on a particular aspect of its environment to the relative exclusion of other aspects. Without such a filtering mechanism, behavior would be completely disorganized since organisms would be continuously responding to trivial as well as important information. It is because of a mechanism such as this that stimulation from our clothing goes without notice. Even the pressure of a belt that is drawn rather tightly will soon go unnoticed unless it is extremely tight. Likewise, the ticking of a clock in a quiet room will eventually go unnoticed, especially if we become preoccupied with some task. Such a reaction to constant stimulation at the behavioral level is called "habituation."

THE MOTOR SYSTEM

Once information has been received from sensory receptors and has been passed along to the CNS, it is then processed even further, and should any action be necessary, impulses are directed at the activation of the effector (motor) organs—the muscles and glands of the body. This results in either the contraction of the skeletal muscles which cause movement, the contraction of the smooth muscles contained in the internal organs, the secretion of the endocrine and exocrine glands, or some combination of these reactions. In the last analysis, behavior is nothing more than the activity of one of these mechanisms. Since it would take us too far afield in this text to discuss in any way the operation of the various glands of the body, this aspect of motor function is not considered any further; instead we will concentrate on the overall activity of the muscle systems of the body.

The mammalian body is composed of three different kinds of muscle tissue. By far the most numerous are the striated or striped muscles, which are attached to the bones and which are responsible for producing movement. About one-half the total weight of the human body is made up of these muscles, which get their name because of the light and dark striations evident when they are examined under a microscope. The second kind of muscle is called smooth or unstriated. These muscles are responsible for the vegetative functions of the body and are found mainly in the visceral organs such as the stomach, intestine, and urinary bladder, and in the blood vessels. The third type of muscle is found in the heart and is called cardiac muscle.

Striated muscle is innervated by peripheral motor neurons at a synaptic point called the neuromuscular or neuromyal junction. This junction occurs between the muscle and the terminal portion of the motor neuron, called the motor end plate, which further branches into complicated structures called sole feet. The space between a sole foot and the muscle fiber is called the synaptic cleft. It is into this synaptic cleft that the sole foot discharges its chemical neurotransmitter in order to cause the muscle to contract. In the case of the striated muscle, this neurotransmitter is acetylcholine.

The sequence of events actually involved in the transmission of impulses from nerves to muscles is similar to that described for the generation of an excitatory postsynaptic potential in a neuron. When a nerve impulse travels down a motor axon it causes the release of acetylcholine from its sole feet. The transmitter then diffuses across the synaptic cleft and causes a depolarization in the muscle fiber by making its membrane more permeable to sodium. This muscle cell depolarization is called an end-plate potential.

The amount of time elapsing from the release of acetylcholine until a muscle response is produced in striated muscle is approximately 2 msec. By contrast, the transmission of impulses from motor neurons to smooth muscle fibers takes about 50 msec from the time the motor neuron discharges its transmitter until a depolarization can be observed, and it takes approximately 100 msec more for the depolarization to reach its maximum.

The structure of the neuromuscular junction in the case of smooth muscle also differs from that of striated muscle. Instead of the end plate found in conjunction with skeletal muscle, the innervation of smooth muscle is with "naked" axon terminals which release their transmitter substances diffusely, thus causing them to spread over more of the muscle fiber. This kind of neuromuscular transmission appears to hold for cardiac muscle as well. Although many of the nerve endings that supply smooth muscle secrete acetylcholine as a neurotransmitter, a few secrete norepinephrine instead. This difference is discussed in more detail when the autonomic nervous system is examined.

When muscles contract, they produce either movement or tension. The tension that is produced in muscles that do not shorten is used to prevent movement, for example, holding a weight in position. The contraction of skeletal muscles is controlled either by reflex or by voluntary activity arising in the brain. Although smooth and cardiac muscle contractions are also regulated by nervous activity, some of these muscles such as the heart still continue to contract rhythmically even when the connections between it and the nerves supplying it have been severed. Because we are not usually aware of the activity of smooth muscles, for example, the beating of the heart or the digestion of food, and because many of the muscles of the visceral organs and heart can contract without nervous stimulation, they are often called involuntary muscles. By contrast, the striated muscles are called voluntary because we are aware of their activity and because they require nervous stimulation to function. However, this distinction is not really valid for several reasons. For one, humans and animals can learn to control many of their visceral muscles, for example, those involved in bowel and bladder function. For another, somatic skeletal muscles often do react without our awareness. The activation of many of our reflexes is one such instance of somatic muscular activity that often occurs without our awareness.

As we have noted already, despite the fact that smooth and cardiac muscles are able to contract automatically, they are still innervated by nerve fibers. The nerves supplying these muscles actually form a special subdivision of the peripheral motor nerve system called the autonomic nervous system (ANS) which itself has two main divisions—the sympathetic and the parasympathetic. These two subdivisions act in opposition. Whereas one system causes excitation, the other causes inhibition. For example, activity in the sympathetic system increases heart rate and slows down the digestive processes in the stomach, whereas parasympathetic activity decreases heart rate and facilitates digestion. In general, the sympathetic system is involved in the mobilization of the body's resources for maximum effort, whereas the parasympathetic system is involved mainly in conserving these resources.

The sympathetic division of the ANS is a two neuron system. The first neuron is called the preganglionic neuron and has its cell body in the spinal cord. Its axon passes out of the cord and synapses with a second neuron, the postganglionic neuron, whose cell body is contained in a grouping of cell bodies that lie alongside the spinal cord, and which together are called the sympathetic chain. The postganglionic axon then passes directly to its target organ.

One of the important target organs activated directly by preganglionic fibers in the sympathetic system, however, is the adrenal gland, which secretes epinephrine into the bloodstream as one of its hormones. Epinephrine itself acts directly on smooth muscle to produce much the same effect as that produced by the sympathetic nerves. In addition, epinephrine increases the activity of the reticular activating system (RAS) (see p. 48), which in turn causes additional firing of the sympathetic nerves. This results in a closed loop circuit: sympathetic activity → adrenal activity (epinephrine) → RAS activity → sympathetic activity. Since the sympathetic system is responsible for producing many of the visceral sensations characteristic of intense emotion ("flight or fight"), this feedback system is conceivably one of the reasons that intense emotional arousal takes so long to disappear after the emotion-producing situation has been removed (Hebb, 1966).

The parasympathetic system also has a preganglionic and postganglionic neuronal link, but unlike the sympathetic system, there is no comparable chain of nerve cell bodies lying outside the spinal cord. Instead, preganglionic fibers in this system pass directly from their cell bodies in the spinal cord to their target organs. They then synapse with their postganglionic fibers either in the vicinity of their target tissue or in the actual walls of the target tissue. Activity in these fibers counteracts that originating in the sympathetic system and tends to restore the vegetative aspects of bodily integrity.

In both the sympathetic and the parasympathetic systems, the preganglionic fibers secrete acetylcholine as their neurotransmitter substance. This is also true of the postganglionic fibers of the parasympathetic system. However, the majority of postganglionic fibers in the sympathetic system have norepinephrine as their neurotransmitter. This is one of the reasons that epinephrine is able to mimic much of the activity of the sympathetic system since in chemical structure, epinephrine resembles norepinephrine.

FUNCTIONAL ORGANIZATION OF THE CNS

The central nervous system is concerned with the integration and control of all bodily activities. It receives signals from the environment, both external and internal, analyzes them, and transmits signals of its own to the various motor structures of the body, the muscles and glands.

Whereas the neuron is the basic functional unit of the nervous system, the reflex is the basic functional unit of behavior. Reflexes represent the simplest pathways by which receptors are connected to effectors in the body. This connection, however, is not direct. Instead, the neuron that carries information from a receptor and the neuron that carries information to an effector are often separated by a third neuron, a centrally connecting internuncial neuron, as it is called, which is located in the spinal cord or in the brain. The simple reflex is thus made up of several basic units: a receptor, which is actually a sensory nerve ending, an internuncial neuron, a motor neuron, and an effector. Reflexes occur at all levels of the spinal cord and the brain and are responsible for many of the bodily functions that go on without our awareness, such as respiration and digestion.

The majority of neural connections in man, however, are much more complex than this simple three chain reflex arc. They tend rather to be comprised of a great many internuncial neurons which link various levels of the spinal cord and brain together. This results in a network in which each sensory neuron is potentially linked through the spinal cord and brain with a rather sizable number of motor neurons. Conversely, each motor neuron is potentially in communication with a great many sensory neurons from all over the body. For its part, the CNS is able to modify reflex activity by sending out impulses which are able to facilitate or suppress activity occurring in the various neuronal pathways that pass through the spinal cord.

One of the reasons that the CNS is able to modify nervous activity in this way is because of the functional organization of the billions of nerve cells of which it is comprised. This organization has been defined in terms of anatomical, cytoarchitectural, neurochemical, and behavioral characteristics. For present purposes, however, four distinct functional-anatomical divisions will be described. These are the spinal cord, the hindbrain, the midbrain, and the forebrain.

A primary function of the spinal cord is to conduct impulses to and from the brain. Sensory impulses from every part of the body except the head travel to the brain through the cord, and similarly, the neural control of all the activities of the body except the head region travel back down through the cord. The spinal cord thus contains the important conduction pathways that mediate sensory and motor activities. In addition to its importance as a conduction pathway, however, the spinal cord also integrates some kinds of information on its own, such as occurs in many of the body's reflexes, for example, the knee jerk.

The hindbrain and the midbrain, which together are known as the brain stem, are basically extensions and elaborations of the spinal cord since many of the ascending and descending fibers which pass through the cord also pass through these areas of the brain. However, in addition to their roles as conduction pathways, the hindbrain and midbrain also perform some important functions of their own. For instance, the medulla, a part of the hindbrain which is located directly above the spinal cord, contains the cell bodies of nerves that regulate such fundamental life processes as breathing, heartbeat, blood pressure, swallowing, and vomiting. Directly above the medulla is the pons, which functions mainly as a transmission center. Directly behind the pons is the cerebellum, which is concerned with the coordination of muscle movements and balance. The cerebellum receives impulses from the motor and sensory areas of the cortex, the inner ear, the muscles, and joints, and through its various connections, it integrates all these impulses in order to synchronize and coordinate bodily movements. The midbrain connects the hindbrain and the diencephalon. It is mainly important as a relay station for visual and auditory input and as such it oversees a number of reflex activities such as blinking, pupillary constriction, and reflex orientation of the head toward the source of auditory stimulation. The two main centers in this area which control these activities are the superior colliculi (vision) and the inferior colliculi (audition).

The forebrain is divided into two main areas, the diencephalon and the telencephalon. The diencephalon consists of the thalamus and the hypothalamus along with several other important structures not discussed here.

The thalamus is an important sensory relay station in the brain. It receives impulses from the various sensory afferent pathways of the body and projects these to specific sensory areas in the cerebral cortex. The thalamus also performs many other functions, some of which involve the regulation of the spontaneous electrical activity characteristic of the cortex (see below).

The hypothalamus is a very small area in the brain, no larger in diameter than a dime. But despite its size, it controls many important bodily functions. For one thing, it oversees the reactivity of the autonomic nervous system since the nuclei in its anterior portion control parasympathetic activity and those in its posterior region control sympathetic activity. As a result, it is able to regulate many of the homeostatic activities of the body. Body temperature, for example, is regulated by causing vasodilation, increasing sweating and respiration, and lowering metabolism when heat loss is necessary. When heat production is required, the opposite effects are produced. In addition, the hypothalamus contains nuclei that are involved in such diverse functions as eating, drinking, sleep, sexual behavior, and emotional reactivity. The hypothalamus also controls the functioning of the 'master gland" of the body, the pituitary, which is located directly below it. The pituitary is called the master gland because its secretions affect the output of many of the other endocrine glands of the body.

The telencephalon, or cerebrum, is composed of two cerebral hemispheres which contain the cerebral cortex and a number of important neural centers and pathways. All the sensory systems of the body project to specific areas of the cortex and many of the nerves controlling the motor system have their cell bodies in this area of the brain as well. In addition, the cerebral cortex contains a large number of cell bodies that are not involved directly in either sensory or motor function. These are the association areas which control the more complex aspects of human behavior.

The cortex itself is divided into four lobes, each of which serves some important sensory, associative, or motor function. The occipital lobes, which are located toward the back of the cerebrum, constitute the primary visual centers. The temporal lobes are located in the region of the temple; they represent the primary auditory centers. In addition, the temporal lobes are involved in speech and memory function. The parietal lobes are located directly in front of the occipital lobes. This is the area to which sensory information from all parts of the body is directed. The frontal lobes, which are located directly in front of the parietal lobes and above the temporal lobes, are involved in the control of voluntary movements as well as some of the complex intellectual functions such as learning and thinking. Two of the important motor pathways that also originate in this area of the brain are the pyramidal and the extrapyramidal systems. The pyramidal system carries impulses from the motor areas of the cortex which initiate movements in the body, especially the skilled movements of the fingers. The extrapyramidal system, on the other hand, regulate the more stereotypical reflex movements of the body.

Another important structure located in the telencephalon is the limbic system. This is a relatively old part of the brain and consists of a number of neural centers such as the hippocampus, the amygdala, and the septum. This system is integrated with parts of the thalamus and the hypothalamus, and it is believed that it is intimately involved in "emotional" behavior. For example, destruction of the amygdala often results in passivity and increased sexual behavior, whereas destruction of the septum often results in a marked increase in aggressiveness. On the other hand, electrical stimulation of parts of this system such as the septum has been shown to have rewarding properties since animals will press a lever for more than 1000 times an hour in order to stimulate this area of the CNS. As a consequence of this phenomenon, this and related areas are sometimes said to contain the "pleasure" centers of the brain.

In addition to these four main divisions, namely, the spinal cord, the hindbrain, the midbrain, and the forebrain, there is another system which consists of interconnected neurons extending from the medulla through the posterior hypothalamus up to the lower thalamus. This diffuse network is known as the reticular activating system (RAS). The RAS receives collaterals from all the sensory pathways except the olfactory, and it sends projections to all the major areas of the cortex. Thus activity in sensory pathways has the effect of arousing the cortex via direct sensory pathways and, indirectly, via activity in the RAS. The RAS, in fact, is directly responsible for the "level of arousal," "generalized drive," "psychic tensions," etc., manifested by an organism at any particular moment. For example, bilateral lesions in this area of the brain will produce permanent coma, even though the sensory pathways to the cortex are left intact. The relationship between the RAS and the various areas of the brain is schematically diagramed in Fig. 1.13.

The electrical activity of the brain can be measured and recorded by means of the electroencephalograph (EEG). This technique uses surface electrodes attached to the scalp to pick up and amplify potential differences in large numbers of cortical cells. These potential differences reflect neural activity at deeper areas of the brain, which manifests itself through the changes produced in the polartiy of cortical cells. When cortical cells change polarity at roughly the same time, synchronized or "relaxed" patterns are produced (see Fig. 1.14). Such patterns, identified as alpha wave activity, have a frequency of 8 to 13 cps. When an individual is alerted, his cortical cells do not change polarity together and as a result, his cortical rhythms become desynchronized or "excited." These patterns, called beta wave activity, have a frequency of about 14 to 40 sec. Conversely, as an individual passes through the various stages of sleep, there is a progressive increase in the amount of theta (4 to 7 cps) and delta ($\frac{1}{2}$ to 3 cps) waves manifested by the EEG (see Fig. 1.15). Not shown in the figure is the "paradoxical" phase of sleep which is characterized by rapid eye movement (REM). The EEG observed under this condition very closely resembles the activity seen during the waking "excited" state.

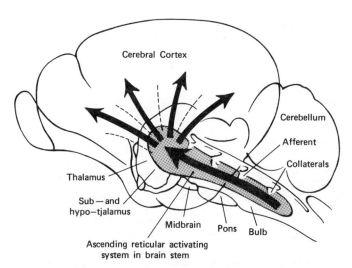

Fig. 1.13 Outline of brain of cat, showing distribution of afferent collaterals to ascending reticular activating system in brain stem (from Starzl et al., 1951).

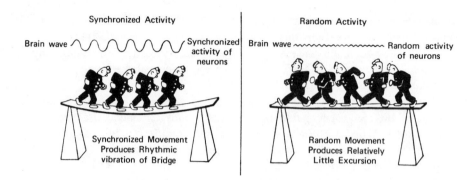

Fig. 1.14 Diagram illustrating on the left how large waves can be built up by synchronized activity of individual neurons (represented by soldiers). On the right, when neurons are not synchronized, little total activity (as represented by the excursion of the bridge) is generated (from Faulconer and Bickford, 1960).

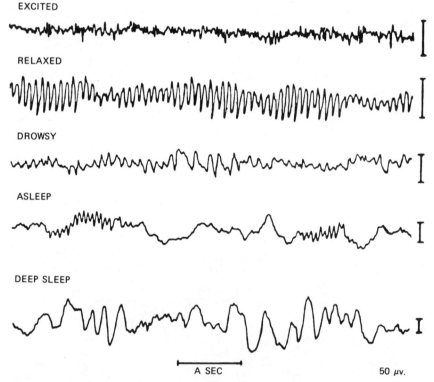

Fig. 1.15 Effect of general excitatory states. Normal electrograms as varied by conditions of generalized excitation, relaxation, drowsiness, light sleep, and deep sleep (from Jasper, 1941).

Because the EEG offers a means of examining neural activity in the brain, it has often been used to observe the gross neural effects of many central acting drugs. As a result of these studies, it has been found that every drug that has some effect on behavior also produces quantitative and qualitative changes in the electrical patterning of the brain. Some of these changes are increases/decreases in the frequency of discharges, in the amplitude of activity, or in the phase relationships between waves (e.g., hypersynchronization or desynchronization); or the appearance of new patterns, for example, sleep, or increased/decreased responsiveness to sensory stimulation. The ability to detect such changes is useful not only for examining the effects of drugs per se, but also for classifying drugs according to their modes of action.

In reviewing the structure and function of cells and the organization of the nervous system, a rather simplistic picture of the machinery of the body has been presented. In so doing, the intention has been not to oversimplify this material, but rather to present an overview that will serve as a base from which to develop the general purpose of this text. Accordingly, in the following chapters, an attempt is made to discuss the effects of drugs in the context of the foregoing presentation.

2. Biological Factors Affecting the Activity of Drugs

Broadly defined, pharmacology is that branch of biology that is concerned with the action of drugs on living systems. The term drug refers to any substance that is used to modify or explore physiological systems or pathological conditions in a living organism. When we speak of neuropharmacology we are referring to that area within pharmacology that is concerned with drugs whose primary site of action is in the nervous system. The term neuropsychopharmacology carries this refinement one step further by restricting the field of inquiry to drugs that act mainly on the central nervous system. It is because this text is devoted primarily to this latter, narrowly defined discipline that Chapter 1 has reviewed the structure, function, and organization of nerve cells in the central nervous system.

A certain familiarity with the structure and function of cells, in fact, is a prerequisite to the study of any branch of pharmacology. Drug action cannot be appreciated adequately without an understanding of the factors that affect the movement of drugs from their sites of administration to the cells on which they act, as well as the reasons for their acting on some cells and not others.

In the case of drugs taken by mouth, for instance, a compound is first swallowed and then goes into the gastrointestinal tract. It must then dissolve in the gastrointestinal fluids before it can pass into the bloodstream. Once it has entered the bloodstream it is distributed to various parts of the body where it may be stored, be transformed, produce a pharmacological effect, or be excreted. Since the blood distributes the drug indiscriminately throughout the body, it may or may not also produce some action on a part of the body in addition to the effects in the CNS for which it was intended, thus causing side effects in addition to its main effect on the brain.

During this movement of a drug from outside an organism to its interior it must traverse several cellular membrane barriers, each of which is surrounded by fluids (see Fig. 2.1). Together, the membranes and these surrounding fluids exert a certain selectivity on the kind of drugs that will be allowed to pass through them. It is only after the membrane containing the drug's receptors has been contacted and the drug has combined with those receptors [the part(s) of the cell with which it interacts to produce its characteristic effects], however, that a drug can be said to have reached its site of action.

In the case of a drug such as aspirin, there is little difficulty in the passage from gastrointestinal tract to the brain. If insulin in introduced into the gastrointestinal tract, however, it will not even pass the first membrane barrier because insulin is acted upon and destroyed by enzymes that are present in the stomach. Therefore, if insulin is taken by mouth, it will have no physiological effect. The examples of aspirin and insulin should thus make evident that without an appreciation of the factors that can affect the activity of drugs from the moment they are taken into the body, it is hardly possible to understand how drugs are able or not able to produce certain effects on behavior. It is only recently, however, that serious research efforts have been devoted to the principles that determine bioavailability, that is, the actual amount of drug available at its receptor sites following administration of a given dose of that drug. This chapter reviews some of

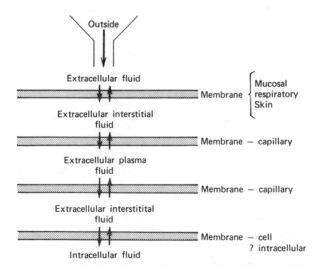

Fig. 2.1 Schematic representation of membranous barriers involved in translocation of a foreign chemical from outside the mammalian organism to intracellular fluid in a tissue cell (from Loomis, 1968).

these principles involving the relationship between the physicochemical characteristics of drugs and their biological actions.

MECHANISMS OF CELLULAR TRANSPORT

The movement of drugs across cell membrane constitutes one of the most important factors determining whether a drug will reach its site of action and hence be in a position to exert a biological response. The passage of drugs across such membranes can occur by means of one or more of the following processes.

Passive Diffusion

As pointed out in Chapter 1, cell membranes are made up largely of protein and lipid material. Because of this structural characteristic, the more soluble a drug is in solvents similar to lipids and protein, the more easily it can traverse cell membranes. Although it is rather difficult to measure the absolute solubility of many compounds since they tend to be extremely soluble in water or organic solvents such as ether and chloroform, a difference in the relative solubility of drugs has been determined by ascertaining how much of a given compound distributes itself between the two phases of a water and lipid mixture. The concentration of the compound in each phase can then be measured and expressed as a ratio. Such ratios are formally referred to as oil/water partition coefficients. The higher the oil/water coefficient of a drug, the greater its degree of lipid solubility, and therefore the greater the ease with which it ought to migrate from the aqueous fluids outside cells into the lipid material contained in cell membranes. Drugs that traverse cellular membranes simply by virtue of their ability to dissolve in the lipid phase of a membrane are said to be transported by passive diffusion.

The actual rate of passive diffusion of a drug across a membrane is described by Fick's law. Without going into the mathematics involved, this law states that the rate of diffusion of a drug is directly proportional both to the surface area of the absorbing membrane and to the difference in the concentration of drug on either side of the membrane, and is inversely proportional to the thickness of the membrane. Thus in addition to the characteristics of the drug and the membrane, the transfer of a drug by diffusion across a cell membrane is similar to the tendency of water to seek its own level. This means that the flow of blood past the site of administration will tend to promote the absorption of a given drug by maintaining a low drug concentration on the plasma side of the membrane opposite to where the drug is highly concentrated.

Filtration

In the case of drugs that are not lipid soluble, some other means besides passive diffusion must exist to facilitate their movement across cell membranes. One such process that is related to passive diffusion with respect to the influence of the concentration gradient is called filtration. If they are small enough, drug molecules that are lipid insoluble (water soluble) may penetrate cellular membranes very rapidly by filtering through the pores of the membrane; the smaller the drug molecule, the more easily and the more quickly it passes from one side of the membrane to the other.

Specialized Transport

To account for the rapid cellular transfer of many large, lipid-insoluble molecules such as the monosaccharides, the concept of specialized "carriers" has been proposed. Two general types of specialized transport mechanisms have been suggested—facilitated diffusion and active transport.

Both these types of transport are believed to involve the movement of substances by "carriers" which are presumed to be associated with specialized components of cellular membranes. It is believed that these "carriers" form complexes with drug molecules on one surface of the membrane, carry them through the membrane, and then dissociate from them on the opposite surface. In the case of facilitated diffusion, this mechanism involves only the movement of drugs from areas of high concentration to those of low concentration. Active transport, on the other hand, involves the movement of drug molecules against the concentration gradient (i.e., from areas of low concentration to areas of high concentration), or in the case of ions, against the electrochemical potential gradient such as is believed to occur in the case of the "sodium pump." The "sodium pump" involves the movement of sodium ions from the inside of the nerve cell to the exterior against a gradient, since the exterior of the nerve cell already contains a great many more sodium ions than are present within the nerve cell. Active transport also differs from facilitated diffusion in requiring a source of energy to function. Hence the active transport mechanism can be inhibited by substances that interfere with cellular metabolism.

Pinocytosis

This involves the surrounding of substances by a portion of the cell membrane, such as occurs in the feeding behavior of the amoeba. Although there is some evidence indicating that pinocytosis can occur in mammalian cells (Lewis, 1937; Holter, 1959), this process is far too slow to be of importance in drug action.

In summary, passive diffusion and filtration are the two main processes by which most drugs appear to move across cellular membranes. The other mechanisms also may be involved in drug transport, but as yet their contribution to the movement of drugs has not been as clearly eluciated. Consequently, most of the following remarks bear mainly on those variables that affect passive diffusion and filtration.

FACTORS AFFECTING DIFFUSION AND FILTRATION

Until psychoactive drugs come into contact with their receptors in the CNS they have no biological effect of their own. The rate of diffusion across a membrane is proportional to the difference in drug concentration on either side of the membrane. Since the blood rapidly distributes drugs throughout the body, the concentration of a drug in the blood in the vicinity of its site of injection will typically be much lower than the concentration of drug at the administration site. Consequently, drugs tend to be absorbed fairly rapidly from various sites of the body.

The peak concentration of a drug that is absorbed into the bloodstream is related closely to the amount of drug present at the site of administration. The higher the drug dosage, the higher ought to be the blood peak level and therefore the faster and more intense ought to be the response to the drug, assuming that the blood levels reflect the relative concentration of drug molecules present at receptor sites. This assumption is based on the principle that the concentration of drug molecules at receptor sites will tend to establish an equilibrium or steady-state condition with the concentration of drug molecules passing through the blood in the area of the receptors.

Since the concentration of a drug at a particular site is a function of its dilution in the fluids at that site, it is obvious that the speed of onset and intensity of the effect produced by a given dose of drug may be affected significantly by the volume of the injection. For instance, a dose of 5 mg/kg of drug X may produce a much greater response if the volume of injection is 0.5 ml/kg than if the volume is 10.0 ml/kg (cf. Warner et al., 1953; Schriftman and Kendritzer, 1957). (See Fig. 2.2.) However, because of their limited solubility, some drugs may be more active when administered in larger rather than small volumes. This is because the process of dissolution has to precede that of absorption, and although a small volume of solvent may facilitate the latter process, it may not be very favorable for facilitating the process of dissolution.

In addition to dosage and volume, the physicochemical properties of a drug constitute an important variable in determining its absorption from its site of administration. We have dealt already with lipid solubility and

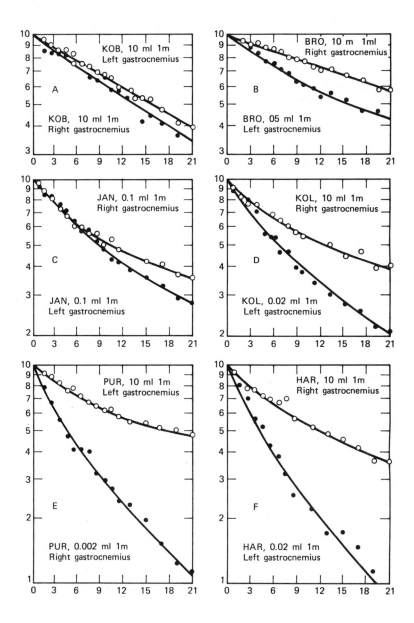

Fig. 2.2 Changes in intramuscular radiosodium clearance rates produced by varying injection volumes in six normal young men. Ordinates are normalized activities in counts per minute. Abscissas are expressed as minutes following injection. The initials of the subject and the volume and site of the injection are indicated on each graph. The smaller the volume, the faster the disappearance ratio (from Warner et al., 1953).

molecular size as being two characteristics of drugs that affect their passage across membranes. We turn now to a related characteristic, namely, the extent of ionization which a drug may undergo when placed in solution.

Most drugs are either weak acids or weak bases which exist in both ionized and un-ionized forms in solution. In simple terms, a drug that has become ionized is one that has split into electrically charged particles. Acids are substances that produce hydrogen ions (H^+), whereas bases are substances that produce hydroxyl (OH^-) ions in aqueous solutions. Since only the unionized form of a drug is lipid soluble, ionization of drugs has important consequences as far as their movement across cellular membranes is concerned.

The extent to which a drug ionizes in solution depends upon its own inherent properties and the hydrogen ion concentration (pH) of the aqueous solution into which it is placed. For example, a drug that is acidic in solution tends to dissociate less if the solution into which it is placed is acidic to begin with. Conversely, a drug that is basic in an aqueous solution ionizes to a much greater extent in an acidic environment. This state of affairs is the exact opposite when the medium into which a drug is placed is basic in nature.

If we consider the fluids of the body essentially as aqueous media separated from one another by membranes, then one way of decreasing the ionization of drugs that are weak acids is to make the solutions into which they are placed more acidic. The less they are ionized, the greater the facility with which they will move across a cellular membrane into the bloodstream. To promote the absorption of drugs that are weak bases, an increase in the basicity of the biological fluids into which they are placed would be required.

The extent to which a drug will behave as an acid or a base is dependent upon its pK_a, which is defined as the pH at which the concentrations of ionized and un-ionized molecules in solution are equal. Mathematically, the relationship between the degree of ionization of a drug (its pK_a) and the pH of its solution is described by the Henderson-Hasselbach equation:

$$pK_a + \log \frac{\text{concentration of ionized drug}}{\text{concentration of un-ionized drug}} = pH$$

If this equation is rearranged to

$$\frac{\text{concentration of ionized drug}}{\text{concentration of un-ionized drug}} = 10^{pH - pK_a}$$

it becomes apparent that a very small change in the pH in the direction of the pK_a can have a considerable effect on the degree of ionization. This is shown in Table 2.1.

Table 2.1   Effect of pH on Ionization of Salicylic Acid
($pK_a = 3.0$)[a]

pH	$pK_a - pH$	Percent Un-ionized
6	-3.0	0.100
5	-2.0	0.990
4	-1.0	9.09
3	0	50.0
2	+1.0	90.9
1	+2.0	99.0

[a] Adapted from Doluisio and Swintosky (1965).

In the stomach, where the pH of the gastric fluids is rather low (pH = 1.4), drugs like the barbiturates which are slightly acidic tend to remain in a relatively un-ionized state; as a result they are readily absorbed from this area. Conversely, drugs that are slightly basic, such as morphine and quinine, tend to ionize in the stomach and as a result they are poorly absorbed from this area. These drugs do not become absorbed until they reach the intestine, which is less acidic than the stomach. The effect of increasing the pH of the biological fluids in the intestine on the absorption of drugs from this area is shown in Table 2.2.

Table 2.2   Effect of Altering the pH of the Intestine in the Rat on the Absorption of Drugs[a]

Drug	pK_a	Absorption (%)			
		pH 4	pH 5	pH 7	pH 8
Salicylic acid	3.0	64	35	30	10
Benzoic acid	4.2	62	36	35	5
Amidopyrine	5.0	21	35	48	52
Quinine	8.4	9	11	41	54

[a] Data are from Brodie (1964).

Table 2.3 illustrates the practical implications of being able to alter the pH of the stomach on the lethality of strychnine (a week base). With the stomach made alkaline by administering sodium bicarbonate, as little as 0.5 mg/kg strychnine is fatal. However, in the normal acidity of the stomach (pH = 2.0) 100 times this amount (50 mg/kg) produces no effect. The reason for this difference in lethality should be readily apparent by now. With the stomach made alkaline, the drug remains relatively un-dissociated and therefore it has no difficulty in crossing the cell membranes of the stomach into the bloodstream. On the other hand, with the stomach slightly acidic, the degree of dissociation is increased markedly and as a consequence so little of the drug is absorbed into the bloodstream that hardly any of the animals are killed.

Table 2.3   Effect of Altering Stomach pH on Lethality of Strychnine Sulfate in the Cat[a]

Dose of Drug (mg/kg)	pH	Time from Injection to Death (minutes)
0.5	8.5	109
1	8.5	48
2	8.5	50
5	8.5	24
10	8.5	24
20	8.5	13
5	1.2	Survived
5	5.8	Survived
10	5.8	Survived
20	1.2	Survived
20	5.8	Survived
50	2.0	Survived
50	5.7	106

[a] Data are from Travell (1940).

In the case of un-ionized molecules, the fact that lipid solubility is the primary variable affecting their absorption across the gastric epithelium is apparent from Table 2.4, which shows the absorption values of three bar-biturate drugs, barbital, secobarbital, and thiopental, which have almost identical pK_a values. The table indicates that thiopental is absorbed very rapidly, secobarbital less so, and barbital hardly at all. These results are directly related to the relative lipid solubility of each drug, thiopental being much more soluble in the oil phase of an oil/water mixture than barbital. Although these data are taken mainly from a study involving the absorption of drugs from the rat stomach (Schanker et al., 1957), data from the human stomach tend to be in very close agreement (cf. Hogben et al., 1957).

The lipid solubility of drugs is a consideration not only in the absorption of compounds from their sites of administration, but also in their absorption from the blood and hence in their actions in the central nervous sys-

Table 2.4   Effect of Drug pK_a and Lipid Solubility on the Absorption of Barbiturates from the Rat Stomach[a]

Drug	pK_a	Oil/Water Partition Ratios	Percent Absorbed in 1 Hour from 0.1 M HCl
Barbital	7.8	0.26	4
Secobarbital	7.9	50.7	30
Thiopental	7.6	63.0	46

[a] Adapted from Schanker et al., 1957; Mark et al., 1958.

tem. For instance, an intravenous injection of 100 mg/kg of thiobarbital in dogs produces an immediate loss of consciousness. With the same dose of barbital, however, dogs do not lose consciousness until approximately 30 minutes after intravenous injection. These effects are directly related to the relative lipid solubility of each drug, thiobarbital being approximately 10 to 11 times more soluble in the oil phase of an oil-water mixture than is barbital (Mark et al., 1958). Thus drugs with a low oil-to-water preference tend to pass more slowly into the brain than do drugs which have a greater solubility in lipidlike substances.

Before this discussion is ended, it should be noted that pH tends to have an opposite effect on the rate of dissolution than it has on the rate of absorption. Whereas a low pH tends to facilitate the absorption of weak acids, it tends to impede their dissolution rate in aqueous media.

However, regardless of the pH of the biological fluids into which they are placed, the sodium and potassium salts of weakly acidic drugs tend to dissolve much more rapidly than comparable free acids. This also holds true for the hydrochloride and other strong acid salts. As a result, drugs given in the form of salts tend to have a much more rapid onset than when administered as the parent drug. For example, whereas 40 mg/kg of secobarbital induces sleep in dogs approximately 23 minutes after oral administration, the same dose of sodium secobarbital induces sleep in dogs within 8 minutes. With the sodium salt, peak blood levels occur within 10 minutes of drug administration whereas with the free acid, peak blood levels do not occur until about 80 minutes after the animals receive the drug (Anderson, 1964).

ROUTES OF ADMINISTRATION

When a drug is inserted into the body, it is generally carried to its site of action through the bloodstream. However, before this is possible, the drug must first be absorbed from the outer side of a cell membrane barrier (unless it is placed directly into the blood; see below). Some of the factors that affect the rate of absorption across cell membranes now have been examined. Since the mechanisms responsible for cell membrane transport are the same for all cells, any differences in the observable rate of the movement of drugs into the bloodstream from their sites of injection must be due to the unique structural features of the cells and the fluids present at the site of administration. This in turn implies that the route by which a drug is administered can have a profound effect on both the degree and the rate of its absorption, as well as on the transformations to which it may be subjected before it finally comes into contact with its receptors.

There are two main routes of drug administration—enteral and parenteral. The enteral route usually means oral administration (per os, p.o.) and generally involves absorption from the gastrointestinal tract. Parenteral routes involve subcutaneous (s.c.), intramuscular (i.m.), intraperitoneal (i.p.), or intravenous (i.v.) injection. There is also the possibility of placing drugs intracisternally (i.c.), that is, directly into the cerebrospinal fluid (CSF), or intraventricularly, which means directly into the ventricular system of the brain. However, except for i.c. spinal anesthesia, the latter two routes are not common methods of administering drugs even in the case of laboratory animals.

The route of administration has a direct bearing on the speed of onset and the intensity of drug action. Since the fluids at various sites in the body are likely to have vastly different pH values, the degree of ionization and hence the rate of movement of a drug into the bloodstream are in large measure responsible for these parameters of drug action.

As noted previously, drugs do not exert pharmacological effects until they are present at their receptor sites at some concentration equal to or greater than necessary to trigger their receptors. Since an equilibrium or steady-state condition tends to become established between the concentration of a drug at its receptors and the concentration of that drug in the bloodstream, there will also be a threshold blood level which corresponds to the threshold level of a drug at its site of action. Hence variations in parameters of drug action such as speed of onset of action and intensity of effect tend to be correlated positively with the concentration of a drug in the blood. The concentration of a drug in the bloodstream is in turn affected by the route by which that drug is administered, for this has a direct bearing on the rate of drug absorption.

Variation in the speed of onset of the drug delta-9-tetrahydrocannabinol (Δ^9-THC), the principal active component in marihuana is depicted in Fig. 2.3 as a function of the route of administration. Pigeons were first trained to peck a key for food reinforcement. Once a stable rate of responding had been established, 10 mg/kg of Δ⁹-THC was administered intravenously, intramuscularly, or orally and the animals were placed immediately into their experimental chambers and their behavior was monitored for the next 2 hours. The figure illustrates that the ongoing rate of key-pecking behavior was suppressed immediately when the drug was administered intravenously, whereas it required approximately 90 minutes for suppression to occur with the same dosage of drug when it was administered intramuscularly. When the drug was given orally, however, no suppression of activity could be discerned.

Fig. 2.4 graphically presents the relationship between the hypothetical blood levels and the onset of action of a drug as a function of different routes of administration. The dotted line represents the threshold concentration necessary to trigger the drug's receptors. The very rapid onset of drug action in case A, which corresponds to intravenous injection, compared with the much slower onset in case B, which represents intramuscular injections, is due to the fact that the threshold drug concentration in the blood is attained much more slowly in the case of the latter route. In case

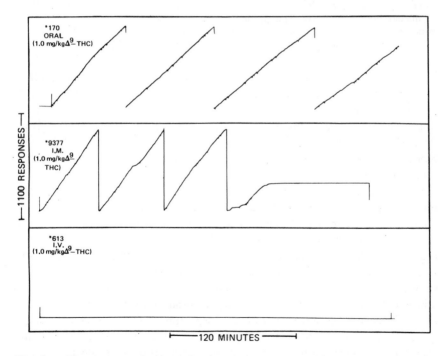

Fig. 2.3 Time-course curves for different routes of administration. Ordinate is rate of key pecking by pigeons working for food reinforcement. Abscissa is time after administration of the drug. See text for further details (from Abel et al., 1974).

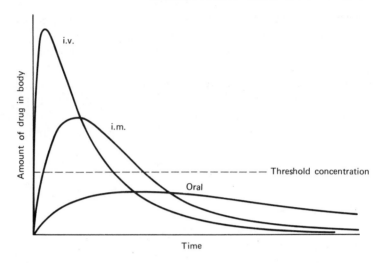

Fig. 2.4 Changes in rate and extent of drug absorption as a function of route of administration. The same dose is given on different occasions. i.v.: drug is absorbed rapidly and completely. This produces a prompt response. i.m.: drug is absorbed completely but more slowly. This produces a delayed and somewhat more prolonged response. Oral: drug is absorbed completely but so slowly that drug levels never reach the threshold level, and therefore dose is ineffective.

C, which corresponds to the oral route, it can be seen that the concentration of drug never rises above the threshold level and no observable effect can be detected.

In addition to the faster onset of action, Fig. 2.4 indicates that a given dose of drug administered intravenously will result in a much higher peak blood concentration than if it is administered by means of some other route. Besides producing a faster onset of action, this ought to produce a much greater suppression of behavior. However, suppression below zero responses per second cannot be demonstrated in the case of Fig. 2.3.

An alternative means of demonstrating that the intravenous route results in a much more intense response involves determining the amount of drug required to kill 50% (LD_{50})* of a given number of animals for each injection route. The results of one such study (Dewey et al., 1971) are shown in Table 2.5. In this experiment, different doses of Δ^9-THC were injected intravenously, intraperitoneally, or orally into rats or mice and the LD_{50}s for each route were determined. Inspection of the table demonstrates quite clearly that with 50% lethality as the criterion, the intravenous route was 2.5 to 5 times more potent than the intraperitoneal route and about 200 to 300 times more potent than the oral route.

* The terms LD_{50} and potency are discussed at much greater length in Chapter 3.

Table 2.5 Lethality of Δ^9-THC in Mice and Rats as a Function of Route of Administration[a]

	LD$_{50}$ (mg/kg)	
Route	Mice	Rats
i.v.	60	97
i.p.	168	560
p.o.	1900	>2000

[a] From Dewey et al. (1971).

In administering drugs for experimental or therapeutic purposes, however, there are often many considerations that determine beforehand which routes of administration can be employed. For example, if a drug precipitates at the pH of blood, it may cause death as a result of embolism. In some situations, there may be a reason for preferring a slow and relatively constant rate of drug absorption rather than a rapid one. Each route of administration obviously carries with it attendant advantages and disadvantages, depending upon the interests of the experimenter or therapist. The following discussion reviews in depth some of the individual problems associated with the various routes of drug administration.

Enteral Routes—Oral (p.o.)

The gastrointestinal tract is the typical route by which drugs are administered to humans. In the case of animals, however, this route is not used as often as are the parenteral routes. The advantages of this route are that it is not painful and, in the case of humans, drugs can be self-administered. For rats and mice, animals that are unable to vomit, the drug is typically injected directly into the oral cavity by means of a needle with a rounded tip. For animals that can vomit, a means by which drugs can be introduced into the gastrointestinal tract is through a tube that is placed into the mouth and then worked gently down the throat almost to the stomach. This method is also used to "force-feed" animals that have been made aphagic with hypothalamic lesions. Administration of drugs by the oral route often is used to obtain parametric information concerning the extent of absorption, the onset and duration of activity, the possible irritant effects of a new drug, etc., all of which are very important factors if a drug is being considered for use in humans.

However, from the point of view of experimental behavioral studies, there are a great many physiological factors associated with the absorption of drugs from the gastrointestinal tract that make it an unreliable route of administration. For one thing, chemical considerations such as the pK_a of a drug and the pH of the biological fluids into which it is placed will be important variables in determining whether the drug will be absorbed at all.

Another important factor to be considered with this route of administration is that drugs that are absorbed from the gastrointestinal tract go directly to the liver. Since the liver is an active site of drug metabolism, the blood level of a drug given in this way may be a great deal lower than if given by one of the other routes of administration.

The presence of food in the stomach is yet another consideration, since food may interfere with the access of a drug to the stomach wall. Food particles may also form an insoluble complex with a drug so that it cannot pass out of the gastrointestinal tract. In addition, a drug may be degraded by enzymes secreted by the stomach in the process of breaking down the food. If drugs are given by the oral route, it is therefore advisable, if not mandatory, to deprive subjects of food for several hours prior to drug administration.

Psychological factors are yet another important source of variability attendant upon oral administration since the "emotional state" of a subject will influence the secretion of enzymes and acids as well as the flow of blood in the area of the gastrointestinal tract. This could markedly affect the reaction to a given drug since the secretion of gastrointestinal fluids could alter the pH of the stomach, thus altering the degree of a drug's ionization; depending on the drug's pK_a, this could either facilitate or interfere with its absorption. An increase in blood flow through this area would, of course, have the effect of increasing the rate of drug absorption.

In summary, there are a great many factors which can affect the absorption of drugs from the gastrointestinal tract so that the oral cavity is not a reliable route of drug administration.

Parenteral Routes

Parenteral injection refers to any route of administration that bypasses the gastrointestinal tract. If the drug remains in solution at its site of injection, it is probable that it will be absorbed fairly rapidly into the bloodstream. On the other hand, since absorption from parenteral sites is influenced by the same physicochemical factors that influence the absorption of drugs from the gastrointestinal tract, there is the possibility that the drug may precipitate due to the pH of the fluids at the site of injection. The peak blood level would then depend upon the rate at which the precipitated drug dissolves back into solution. In general, however, a more rapid rate of onset and a more predictable response effect typically are obtained when drugs are administered by this route than when given enterally. Other advantages attendant upon this route of administration are an opportunity to introduce drugs into the body which would be absorbed poorly if given orally, or which might be metabolized by the liver before reaching their sites of action. Specific advantages and disadvantages connected with each of the various individual parenteral injection routes are outlined below.

SUBCUTANEOUS INJECTION (S.C.)

This method involves injecting a drug directly under the skin. Relatively constant rates of drug absorption can be achieved with this route but the actual speed of absorption varies as a function of the vehicle in which the drug is dissolved, the area over which the solution spreads, and the rate of blood flow in the vicinity of the drug. To obtain a slow reliable rate of absorption from subcutaneous sites, drugs are sometimes implanted under the skin in the form of compressed pellets. Inserting such pellets is a relatively simple procedure for animals such as the mouse. The subject is lightly etherized (chloroform should be avoided since it produces renal damage in mice), a fold is made in the skin above the neck, and an incision is made. The pellet is then inserted in the incision and moved toward the back of the animal. If the mouse is kept in isolation and the incision is small enough so that there is not much bleeding, the wound need not be stitched closed. The ideal shape for such pellets is a flat disc, since the exposed area will diminish only slightly as the disc becomes thinner, thus ensuring a relatively constant level of the drug in the bloodstream.

The rate of absorption from subcutaneous sites can vary greatly, however, depending on such factors as the anatomical region into which the injection is made and the age of the subject being treated.

With regard to the former variable, an experiment reported by Nora et al. (1964) involved a comparison of the rate of absorption of radioactively labeled insulin from subcutaneous arm and thigh injections in humans. The results showed that when the drug was injected under the skin of the arm, its mean absorption half-life was 224 minutes as compared to 310 minutes for the subcutaneous thigh injection. A difference of this magnitude, the investigators point out, could be an important factor in diabetic control.

The effects of age on the absorption of drugs from a subcutaneous site were reported by Lee (1966) using chlorpheniramine maleate and diphenhydramine hydrochloride, two antihistamine drugs. The subjects were rats and the dependent variable was the LD_{50}. During the first 16 days of life, the LD_{50} for chlorpheniramine was between 175 and 230 mg/kg. After the rats were 25 days old, the LD_{50} was 360 to 365 mg/kg. A similar trend was observed for diphenhydramine. No apparent difference between the two age groups was evident in their liver enzyme activity which could account for this result. Another alternative that has been suggested was that the higher LD_{50}s of the older animals were due to a decrease in the amount of drug absorbed from the subcutaneous region. The reasons for such a difference in absorption rate are not readily apparent, but one possibility is that because of the different ages of the subjects, the chemical composition of the subcutaneous tissue may have been different. If there were differences in the fat composition of the cells, for instance, then one might expect a concomitant difference in the oil/water partition coefficient of drugs and therefore an attendant difference in absorption rate (Ballard, 1968).

Other disadvantages of this route of administration worth considering are that some drugs such as alcohol are highly irritating if given subcutaneously and that those which are dissolved in an oily solvent may be absorbed poorly. As a result, peak blood levels may not become high enough to produce any observable response unless a very large dosage of drug is injected.

INTRAMUSCULAR INJECTION (I.M.)

In administering drugs by this route, the needle is placed within the skeletal muscles. Before the injection is actually given, however, the plunger of the syringe should be pulled back to make sure that the needle has not entered a blood vessel.

As in the case of subcutaneous injections, the anatomical region into which a drug is directed via the muscles can also affect the rate of its absorption. For example, the mean absorption half-life for insulin following intramusclar arm injections was found to be 224 minutes as compared with 314 minutes for intramuscular thigh injections (Nora et al., 1964).

In general, absorption from muscle tissue tends to be fairly rapid if the drug is dissolved in an aqueous vehicle. Drugs that are dissolved in oily vehicles, however, may form "depots" at the injection site, this will have the effect of slowing the rate of entry of the drug into the circulation. In addition, drugs such as alcohol may not be suitable for intramuscular injection because of their highly irritant effects.

One factor that warrants consideration if drugs are to be administered intramuscularly is the possibility that muscular exercise will influence the rate of absorption of drugs from these sites. For example, Wisham et al.

(1951) injected radioactively labeled sodium into the biceps muscle of human volunteers. The subjects were then asked either to rest or to lift a 5 lb weight a number of times. The flow of blood and lymph through the biceps muscle was augmented markedly by the exercise, with the result that there was a 100% increase in the rate of disappearance of radioactivity in the exercise condition compared with the rest condition.

A somewhat related study was reported by Barnes and Trueto (1941). These investigators studied the lethality of a number of toxins in rabbits, some of whom were immobilized. Their dramatic results are presented in Table 2.6.

Table 2.6 Effect of Immobilization on Lethality of Tiger Snake Venom, Diphtheria Toxin, and Tetanus Toxin in Rabbits[a]

	Survival Time after Injection into Leg			
	Freely mobile	Number of animals	Immobilized	Number of animals
Tiger snake venom	20 minutes	1	8 hours	6
	60 minutes	1	24 hours	3
	150 minutes	1	Survived	6
Diphtheria toxin	28 hours	1	28 hours	1
	36 hours	1	84 hours	2
	40 hours	2	128 hours	1
			Survived	1
Tetanus toxin	2 days	1	5 days	1
	3 days	2	9 days	2
	4 days	2	11 days	1
	5 days	1	14 days	1
			22 days	1

[a] Data are from Barnes and Trueto (1941).

Likewise, Irwin et al. (1958) have reported that stimulant drugs such as methamphetamine raise the activity levels of rats with normally high levels of activity to a much greater extent than is the case for rats whose normal activity levels are much lower prior to injection. Similarly, depressant drugs such as pentobarbital and chlorpromazine have a much greater depressant effect on the more active animal.

Since animals such as the mouse and the rat are much more active at night than during the day, the time of day at which a drug is administered could be another important factor affecting absorption. On the basis of the three previously mentioned studies, one might predict that excitatory and depressant drugs should produce a much greater effect on the activity levels of rodents if administered during the night than during the day, since the rate of blood flow through muscle tissue ought to be greater during the night resulting in a faster rate of absorption. Much more will be said regarding the interaction of time and drug action when the topic of chronopharmacology is discussed.

A final consideration worth noting is that following a period of exercise, drugs may be absorbed from muscle sites much more rapidly than if they are administered after a period of rest. This observation emerges from a study by Wisham et al. (1951). Compared with the disappearance of radioactively labeled sodium from muscle that had not been exercised, the rate of disappearance from muscle tissue previously fatigued was much faster. This observation may have important implications for animal experiments since in many cases, the subjects are often not gentled prior to drug treatment. Since it is well known that animals such as the rat may react rather violently to being handled for the first time, producing thereby attendant changes in heart rate (Black et al., 1964), it may be advantageous to "tame" such animals prior to drug treatment by subjecting them to frequent handling experiences designed to habituate them to such treatment (Abel, 1971).

INTRAPERITONEAL INJECTION (i.p.)

Although rarely done with humans, the injection of drugs into the peritoneal cavity is probably the most commonly used route in animal laboratory experiments. Drugs are usually taken up very rapidly from the peritoneal cavity into the bloodstream, but again, drugs dissolved in oily vehicles may be absorbed much more slowly than those in aqueous solutions. In general, however, the absorption of drugs from this area tends to be slightly more rapid than absorption from subcutaneous or intramuscular sites regardless of the drug vehicle. Another consideration is that larger volumes of injection can be administered intraperitoneally than with the other two routes without producing untoward side effects.

One of the problems associated with intraperitoneal injections, particularly if they are given to the same animal over a long period of time, however, is the possibility of infection. One way of minimizing this possibility is to inject the drug into different quadrants of the peritoneal cavity.

INTRAVENOUS INJECTION (i.v.)

By placing the drug directly into the bloodstream a very rapid onset of action can be produced. Moreover, the concentration of drug initially available to the blood is known. Other advantages of using this route are that large volumes of drug can be given if the rate of injection is slow, and that drugs that may be highly irritating if given by some other route can often be administered in this manner without the ensuing irritation. Two additional advantages of this route are that it can be used to administer drugs that are poorly absorbed from other sites and that it can be used to administer drugs that might be metabolized before reaching their sites of action (see below).

There are several disadvantages in administering drugs by this route, however. If given too quickly, the injection may produce undesirable cardiovascular and respiratory effects (e.g., sharp decreases in blood pressure or shallow and irregular breathing). Special dangers are also associated with the possible entry of air into the blood. In addition, drugs that are dissolved in oily solvents or those administered as suspensions often cannot be given by this route because of the possibility of embolism (obstruction of blood vessels). If drugs are to be given over a long period of time, chronic intravenous injection may cause damage to the veins resulting in leakage of the drug into surrounding subcutaneous and muscle tissue.

INTRAVENTRICULAR AND INTRACISTERNAL INJECTION

These routes involve placing the drug directly into the brain or the spinal fluid, respectively. Many drugs that are entirely unable to penetrate the brain or else penetrate it to only a limited extent because of the "blood-brain barrier" (see below) may be examined for their direct central effects if given in this manner. In addition, if drugs are given by these routes, it is then possible to contrast their central effects with their combined peripheral and central effects when administered in the conventional manner, for example, subcutaneously or intramuscularly. For example, if injected by a conventional route, epinephrine has an excitatory effect on mammals whereas placement of this chemical directly into the cerebral ventricles induces a sleeplike state resembling light anesthesia (cf. Feldberg and Sherwood, 1954). Finally, by administering drugs to a restricted area of the brain, neuroanatomical sites at which a particular drug is active may be specified more precisely.

However, there are many technical difficulties associated with the administration of drugs in this manner. In addition to damaging the neural tissue through which the cannula must pass, volumes of injection greater than 10 μl into brain tissue may produce lesions that are even larger than those produced by the cannula itself. The size of such lesions is related not only to the injection volume, but also to the number of injections, which makes the results of chronic intracerebral studies very problematical (Rech and Domino, 1959). Besides lesions, mechanical displacement of nerve fibers may also occur if injection volumes are too great (MacLean, 1957). The distribution of drugs from their administration sites is another problem to be considered. Although drugs are often administered intraventricularly to restrict their effects to circumscribed regions of the brain, this purpose often is frustrated by diffusion of a drug away from its injection site. This is very likely if the volume of injection is greater than 20 μl. With volumes of 100 μl, drugs will completely fill one ventricular area and will overflow into another (McCarthy and Borison, 1966, 1967). For this reason, many experimenters (e.g., Grossman, 1962a, 1962b) prefer to administer drugs in solid crystalline form in animal studies involving the placement of drugs into the brain.

For a more detailed discussion of the problems involved in administering drugs intraventricularly and intracisternally, the interested reader should consult the excellent article by Rech (1968).

VEHICLE CONSIDERATIONS

The solvent in which a drug is dissolved or suspended is termed the vehicle. To be suitable for experimental study or therapeutic usage, a vehicle should have no intrinsic activity of its own. Unfortunately, this is not always the case. Since some drugs are soluble only in certain vehicles and since these vehicles do have physical and chemical properties of their own, there are a number of considerations to be entertained in choosing a suitable vehicle for a drug. For example, a drug may be insoluble in a particular vehicle; it may react with the vehicle to form a new compound; the vehicle may have actions of its own which mask, increase, or decrease the effects of the drug; the vehicle may affect the rate of absorption of a drug; the vehicle may be unsuitable for intravenous injection because of the possibility of embolism; finally, a vehicle may be unsuitable simply because of its toxicity.

One of the early studies dealing with the influence of vehicles on drug action examined the effects of sodium pentobarbital and metrazol on the loss of the righting reflex and the production of convulsions, respectively, in mice as a function of the vehicle used to administer these drugs (Hazelton and Hellerman, 1946). The drugs were administered either orally or intravenously and the ED_{50} (effective dose for 50% of the animals) was ascertained for each drug when dissolved in distilled water. The influence of various vehicles was then determined and the effects were expressed in terms of percentage of drug effect compared to when water was the vehicle. The results for sodium pentobarbital are presented in Table 2.7. These data indicate quite clearly that the vehicle in which a drug is dissolved or suspended can contribute greatly to the differences in drug effects.

Table 2.7   Influence of Vehicle on Loss of Righting Reflex in Mice Produced by Sodium Pentobarbital[a]

Vehicle	Route	Dose (mg/kg)	Concentration (%)	Loss of Righting Reflex (%)
Water	Oral	50		52
Propylene glycol	Oral	50	10	48
			25	85
Glycerin	Oral	50	10	38
			25	5
Water	i.v.	30		58
Propylene glycol	i.v.	30	10	65
			25	100
Glycerin	i.v.	30	10	90
			25	100

[a] Adapted from Hazelton and Hellerman, 1946.

Since a large percentage of the body's fluids is water, the solubility of a drug in water often promotes its absorption if the molecule is small enough that it can pass through membrane pores. However, there are certain vehicles that promote drug absorption even more than water. For example, both dimethyl sulfoxide (DMSO) and ethyl alcohol have been shown to increase the penetration of epinephrine (E) and norepinephrine (NE) into the central nervous system of chicks (Hanig et al., 1971, 1972). Representative data for DMSO are presented in Table 2.8.

Table 2.8   Passage of Epinephrine (E) and Norepinephrine (NE) into the Brains of Neonatal Chicks as a Function of Vehicle[a]

Treatment	Amount of E or NE in Brain (μg/g brain weight)	Change (%)
E (in NaCl)	0.38	—
E (in NaCl + DMSO)	0.53	34.8
NE (in NaCl)	0.61	—
NE (in NaCl + DMSO)	0.85	38.8

[a] Data are from Hanig et al. (1971).

In the experiment from which these data are taken, 5 mg/kg of epinephrine or norepinephrine was dissolved either in 0.9% physiological saline (NaCl) or in 50% DMS0 and 0.9% NaCl, and the drugs were then administered intravenously in one of these forms to baby chicks. A few minutes later, the animals were sacrificed and the amounts of epinephrine and norepinephrine present in the brains of these animals were determined. The data indicate that DMS0 increased the epinephrine concentration in the brain by 34.8% and the norepinephrine concentration by 38.8% (Hanig et al., 1971). Alcohol, on the other hand (not shown in table), was found to increase E levels by 28.9% and NE levels by 21.9% (Hanig et al., 1972). Thus these vehicles unquestionably affect the penetration of chemical substances dissolved in them into the brain. This in turn can have important ramifications for drug action. For example, the toxicity of quaternary ammonium compounds in mice and rats is markedly increased when they are dissolved in DMSO (Rosen et al., 1965), even though these compounds hardly pass into the brain at all following systemic injection in other vehicles.

DISTRIBUTIONAL FACTORS AFFECTING DRUG ACTION

The absorption of a drug from the blood to its cellular site of action is governed by many of the same factors that are responsible for its initial movement from its site of injection, for example, lipid solubility, molecular size, and degree of ionization. Since the blood services all the tissues of the body, this means that any drug that is present in the bloodstream will be carried to all parts of the body. And just as the extent of blood flow to a particular area of the body affects the absorption of drugs from that site into the blood, so too does the blood supply to various tissues affect the passage of drug from the blood into a given area. Among those areas that are richly supplied with blood capillaries which may thus be rapidly infused by drugs are the brain, the liver, the kidney, and of course, the heart. Areas that are poorly supplied with blood capillaries are fat, skin, and muscle. This means that drugs will tend to appear in significant concentrations in such areas as the brain long before they enter the fatty tissues of the body.

However, whereas some drugs remain relatively free in the blood, others tend to become bound to substances therein (see below), or are stored in certain bodily tissues with the result that the concentration of free drug relative to its primary receptor sites is significantly reduced. Although the complexes formed between drugs and substances in the blood can also be regarded in terms of drug-receptor interactions, these reactions do not produce any biological effects and therefore they are referred to commonly as sites of loss. The most important sources of these "sites of loss" affecting the activity of drugs are now reviewed.

Protein Binding

Once they enter the bloodstream, many drugs often become "bound" to plasma proteins. The protein material most often involved in such binding is albumin, but binding may also occur with plasma globulins. Since only drugs that are not bound are able to pass through the cellular membranes of the body (Brodie and Hogben, 1957), protein binding emerges as an important variable reducing the amount of active drug in the bloodstream. This in turn also has the effect of reducing the concentration gradient responsible for the movement of a drug from the bloodstream into the cells of the body.

Not all drugs are bound to plasma proteins with the same strength, however. Table 2.9 shows that whereas warfarin and phenylbutazone are almost completely bound to human plasma protein, only about 2% of the absolute amount of barbital is bound in this manner. Moreover, binding is a reversible process. When the concentration of a drug in the blood decreases, the amount of drug previously rendered inactive because of binding now becomes available for entry into bodily cells. Consequently, although protein binding may act to remove a portion of a drug from free circulation, it may also serve to prolong the duration of action of that drug, since drug molecules will move back into free circulation from binding sites as the blood levels decreases due to drug metabolism and/or excretion. This will have the effect of creating more free drug to interact with receptor sites.

The fact that drugs that are bound to protein are rendered pharmacologically inactive has prompted some investigators (e.g., Gibaldi, 1971)

Table 2.9 Percentage of Protein Binding of Drugs in Human Plasma[a]

Drug	Mean Percentage Bound
Phenylbutazone	98
Warfarin	97
Papaverine	90
Thiopental	75
Pentobarbital	40
Tetracycline	35
Ampicillin	15
Barbital	2

[a] Data are from Calesnick (1971).

to question the advisability of using plasma levels of drugs as a basis for comparing drug effects across species as advocated by Brodie (Brodie and Reid, 1972). However, it should be pointed out that protein binding affects the intensity of drug responsiveness only when the concentration of a drug in the blood is quite low to begin with. When peak blood levels are relatively high, the number of binding sites becomes quickly saturated. Although the amount of drug bound to plasma protein may then be at a maximum, the actual percentage of drug bound in this way is usually negligible in comparison with the total amount of drug that is free to diffuse across cell membranes. With a low concentration of drug, however, the proportion of free drug to bound drug tends to approach equality, and with less and less drug, more of it may be bound to plasma protein than is free to diffuse out of the circulation into bodily tissues (cf. Goldbaum and Smith, 1954). What this means, therefore, is that where binding is a possibility, more drug must be administered in order to saturate the various sites of loss so that there will be enough free drug available to its sites of action. Only after this precaution has been taken can species differences in responsiveness to drugs be compared on the basis of blood levels of given compounds. However, this can still become rather complicated because of differences between species in the extent to which they bind protein in the bloodstream. The early research in this area has been thoroughly reviewed by Goldstein (1949). More recent cross-species comparisons of drug binding are reported in the studies of Anton (1960), Borga et al. (1968), and Sturman and Smith (1967). The use of blood levels of drugs to compare species differences in responsiveness to drugs (Brodie and Reid, 1972) is thus not without certain inherent encumbrances.

Directly related to the topic of protein binding is the problem of drug interaction. For instance, if two drugs compete for the same binding sites, the drug with the higher affinity for plasma protein will displace the other. This results in an increase in the concentration of free drug for the latter, thus possibly enhancing its pharmacological activity (cf. Hartshorn, 1970; Gibaldi, 1971). For example, if drug X which is normally 99% bound to plasma protein is displaced somewhat by drug Y so that X is only 95% bound, the amount of drug X now available to interact with its receptors is increased fivefold. This change could significantly increase the toxicity of a hitherto nontoxic chemical (cf. Stockley, 1972).

Localization of Drugs in Bodily Tissue

Many lipid-soluble drugs have an affinity for fat-containing cells. The absorption of such drugs by fatty tissues will have the effect of reducing their blood concentration and hence possibly their pharmacological activity. For instance, thiopental is an anesthetic drug which in small doses has a fast onset and a relatively short duration of action. Within minutes of intravenous administration, the concentration of thiopental in the brain increases greatly, thus accounting for its rapid onset of action. However, just as rapidly, the tissue levels in the brain decline and the drug's anesthetic action is lost. The reason for this relatively short duration of action is that the drug tends to accumulate in the fatty tissues of the body, causing the drug to be removed from the bloodstream. This in turn causes the drug to move out of the central nervous system due to the lowered concentration of drug in the blood relative to the brain. As a result, the anesthetic activity of the drug is terminated (Brodie et al., 1952). However, if the equilibrium concentrations of thiopental between the blood and the brain were rather high, such as would occur following administration of a large dose of thiopental, this level would then be maintained for a long time because of the brain's saturation by the drug. The period of anesthesia would then be greatly extended (Brodie et al., 1952).

Blood-Brain Barrier

The extent to which a drug leaves the bloodstream to enter the brain depends upon many of the same factors that affect the penetration of drugs through biological membranes in general, for example, lipid solubility, ionization, concentration in the blood, molecular size, the rate of blood flow through a particular area of the brain, degree of plasma binding, and the permeability of the capillaries of the brain for the particular drug. The concept of a "blood-brain barrier" that selectively screens substances from entry into the central nervous system has arisen from the fact that a great many drugs fail to enter brain tissue or cerebrospinal fluid, although they pass with relative ease into other tissues of the body.

The first experiments to investigate the existence of the blood-brain barrier involved the intravenous injection of certain acidic dyes such as trypan blue which were found to stain most bodily organs but left the central nervous system relatively uncolored. Since the areas stained by the dyes did not extend beyond the capillary endothelium of the brain, the blood-brain barrier was proposed to exist at the level of the capillaries of the central nervous system.

These early experiments using vital dyes to study the phenomenon of the blood-brain barrier did not go without criticism, however. Arguments against them ranged from the failure to take into consideration the affinity of dyes for plasma protein and the possible ionization of the dye, which would tend to reduce the amount of free drug available for diffusion into the brain, to the possibility that the dyes might have become discolored by metabolic processes in brain tissue, thus rendering such experiments indecisive (cf. Goldstein et al., 1969).

The first two criticisms, however, could have been applied equally to the entry of these dyes into other bodily tissues which did become stained. The remaining criticism ignored the fact that when these dyes were placed directly into the brain, the areas affected did become stained as well.

The approach was therefore sound after all. The real objection was that these studies were purely qualitative (Bakay, 1957) and therefore indicated nothing about the blood-brain barrier except that it appeared to exist.

In one of the first quantitative studies to be conducted in this area, Wallace and Brodie (1939) administered bromide, iodide, or thiocyanate either orally or intravenously to dogs and compared the amounts of these substances in different tissues at various times after injection. Uptake into the brain was found to be significantly depressed compared to the uptake of these substances into other bodily tissues. More recently, Kleeman et al. (1962) compared the penetration of radioactively labeled urea into the brain cerebrospinal fluid and muscle tissue of rabbits. Urea is a nonpolar, un-ionized, substance and as such, it ought to have penetrated the cellular membranes of the body with relative ease. Although this was shown to be true for muscle tissue, the amount of urea to enter the cerebrospinal fluid was found to be reduced markedly by comparison.

The general view of Brodie and his associates (Brodie et al., 1957) is that the blood-brain barrier acts as a lipoid membrane which permits the passage of drugs in accord with the same factors that govern the passage of drugs from the stomach or intestine. Table 2.10, which is taken from one

Table 2.10 Relationship between Drug Penetration into the Cerebrospinal Fluid and Oil/Water Partition Coefficient[a]

Drug	Protein Binding (%)	pK_a	Undissociated at pH 7.4 (%)	Oil/Water Partition Coefficients (in Chloroform)	Permeability Coefficient
Aniline	35	4.6	99.8	17	0.69
Aminopyrine	12	5.1	99.5	73	0.69
4-Aminoantipyrine	15	4.1	99.9	15	0.69
Antipyrine	2	1.4	99.99	28	0.21
Acetanilide	2	1.0	99.99	3	0.039
N-Acetyl-4-amino-antipyrine	1	0.5	99.99	1.5	0.0051
Thiopental	75	7.6	61.3	102	0.69
Barbital	10	7.8	71.5	2	0.029
Salicylic acid	70	3.0	0.01	0.2	0.0026

[a] Data are from Mayer et al. (1957).

of their studies, contains some of the data upon which they base their hypothesis. These observations were obtained with dogs after enough drug had been administered to ensure complete saturation of binding sites.

Aniline, aminopyrine, 4-aminoantipyrine, and antipyrine are relatively lipid soluble and remain virtually undissociated at the pH of blood (7.4). Consequently, they enter the cerebrospinal fluid rather rapidly. Acetanilide and N-acteyl-4-aminoantipyrine also are almost completely undissociated at pH 7.4, but they are much less lipid soluble and therefore they penetrate the cerebrospinal fluid at a slower rate. The comparison between barbital and thiopental is also illuminating. Both drugs remain undissociated to relatively the same extent, but barbital is much less lipid soluble and therefore it penetrates into the cerebrospinal fluid much more slowly than thiopental. Finally, salicylic acid, which is both poorly lipid soluble and highly ionized, penetrates the most slowly of all.

From these data, it would appear that the penetration through the blood-cerebrospinal fluid boundary of most undissociated drugs is correlated closely with their oil/water partition coefficients (the ratio of the concentration of drug in the lipid phase to its concentration in the aqueous phase of a two-phase system), a situation roughly parallel to the absorption of such drugs from the gastrointestinal tract. The rate-limiting factor for the passage of drugs across this barrier system would thus seem to be the lipid solubility of a compound (Schanker, 1964).

Further evidence that the blood-brain and blood-cerebrospinal fluid barriers are highly resistant to penetration by free organic ions is provided by studies of the movement of completely ionized substances such as quaternary ammonium compounds which traverse these barriers much more slowly than do lipid soluble un-ionized molecules (Brodie et al., 1960; Mayer and Bain, 1956). However, if the dosage of these ionized drugs is large enough, they too may enter the brain to a certain extent as a result of the increased concentration gradient (Mayer and Bain, 1956).

On the other hand, it must be remembered that glucose, which has a very low partition coefficient, is readily able to penetrate the blood-brain barrier, a situation not without importance since the brain relies upon glucose as its main source of metabolic energy. The entry of glucose into the brain suggests that some kind of specialized carrier system must exist by which it and the various other sugars and amino acids are transported into the brain. Should a drug resemble these substances in structure, it would then be possible for it to be transported across the blood-brain barrier in spite of what might otherwise be considered unfavorable physicochemical properties (cf. Brodie, 1964).

The blood-brain barrier is not equally efficient throughout the central nervous system, however; this is evident from the fact that drugs do not penetrate all regions of the brain to the same extent or at the same rate. For example, systemic administrations of norepinephrine penetrate only into the hypothalamus. Other parts of the brain are relatively impermeable to this compound (Weil-Malherbe et al., 1961).

Using radioactively labeled phenobarbital, Domek et al. (1960) determined the amount of radioactivity in various parts of the cat brain $\frac{1}{2}$ and 6 hours after an i.p. injection of this compound. One-half hour after injection, there was a distinct contrast in the amount of radioactivity in the white and gray matter of the central nervous system, the quantity being greatest in the gray. By 6 hours, however, the difference between these two areas had been reduced markedly. Domek et al. surmised that these differences arose because the thick layer of lipoid membranes making up the myelin hindered the entry of phenobarbital into these fibers, compared with their entry into the unmyelinated fibers constituting the gray matter of the brain.

The development of techniques that permit quantitative analysis of the amount of drug localized in different regions of the brain has thus provided further insight into the nature of the blood-brain barrier. Using such techniques, it also has become possible to determine specific anatomical regions of the brain that are penetrated by drugs more readily than others. In one such experiment, Roth et al. (1959) examined the entry of the anticonvulsant drug acetazoline into the brains of cats. They found that in those regions of the brain closest to the cerebrospinal fluid, for example, the hypothalamus, the rate of entry was much faster and the concentration of drug significantly greater than in other regions of the brain. This observation again suggests that the blood-brain barrier prohibits the entry of drugs into some areas of the brain more efficiently than into other areas.

Before we leave the topic of the blood-brain barrier, it should be pointed out that the same principles which apply to the entry of drugs into the central nervous system seem also to apply to their exit (Brodie and Hogben, 1957). Changes in lipid solubility, ionization, pH, etc., are thus of importance at each stage in the activity of drugs.

TERMINATION OF DRUG ACTION

Drugs cease to exert pharmacological effects when their blood concentrations are reduced to subthreshold levels. In general, the rate at which this occurs is related to the amount of drug actually present in the body at any given time. This rate usually is expressed as the biological half-life of the drug and is defined as the time it takes the body to eliminate by means of metabolism and/or excretion one-half the amount of drug initially administered to the organism. Calculation of this half-life value is readily achieved by administering a given amount of drug to the subject and then taking samples of its blood at various times after injection. The blood is then analyzed for drug concentration and these concentrations are plotted against time. The half-life can then be determined by extending a line from the 50% value on the ordinate to the function, and then projecting a perpendicular line from this point to the abscissa (time). The half-life value can then be read from the point of intersection of the perpendicular and the abscissa (See Fig. 2.5).

Should the mechanisms of biotransformation and/or excretion become inoperative, however, drug effects could conceivably go on for a long time (since the blood levels would not be diminished greatly), or at least until the cells responding to a drug became exhausted. The mechanisms and factors responsible for the termination of drug action are thus additional considerations in understanding the activity of drugs.

Biotransformation

One way in which the activity of a drug may be terminated is by altering its physical and/or chemical properties. The chemical reactions involved in such biotransformations generally involve one or more phases (see Williams, 1971). In Phase I, drugs are subjected to one of three major chemical reactions: oxidation, reduction, or hydrolysis. Details of these transformations can be found elsewhere (e.g., DiPalma, 1971; Goodman and Gilman, 1970). The general effect of these transformations is that the polarity of the drug is increased. Such changes tend to make a drug less lipid soluble, which usually translates into a decrease in pharmacological activity. In some cases, however, a drug may be an inactive precursor or "prodrug," which when metabolized becomes more active than the parent compound. One such example is the drug chloral hydrate and its metabolite trichloroethanol. Alternatively, a pharmacologically active drug such as codeine may have a metabolite such as morphine which is also active.

Phase II in the biotransformation of drugs involves a "synthetic" or conjugation reaction which is sometimes described as "detoxication." This term is appropriate, however, only if a drug metabolite is pharmacologically less active and less toxic than its parent compound. Typically, conjugation reactions involve the combination of a drug with substances in the body such as glucuronic acid, a combination which tends to increase the polarity of the metabolite even more.

For the most part, most of the metabolic transformations to which drugs are subjected do not occur spontaneously. Instead they are mostly catalyzed reactions, catalysis being an acceleration of a chemical reaction by some substance which does not undergo any permanent chemical change

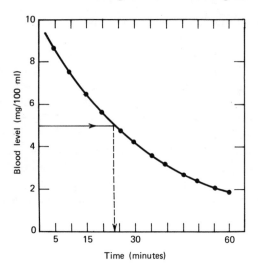

Fig. 2.5 Estimation of biological half-life (see text).

itself. The catalysts of chemical reactions such as those involved in drug metabolism are the enzymes. The reaction between an enzyme and its substrate involves two basic steps. The first is the combination of the substrate and the enzyme to form an intermediate substance known as an enyzme-substrate complex. This intermediate complex then generates a product plus the original enzyme.

In drug metabolism, many of the enzymatic transformations which occur in the body take place in the microsomal endoplasmic reticulum of the liver. Metabolic transformations can occur at other sites as well, but they have not been studied in as much detail. From a pharmacological standpoint, the main effect of the liver microsomal enzyme is that they act upon substances with high lipid solubility and the metabolites resulting from such reactions are generally less lipophilic than the original compound (substrate).

Some of the problems that make generalizations regarding drug effects from animals to man rather tentative, however, are that the concentration of enzymes in various tissues is different across species (see Table 2.11) and that drugs may be metabolized via different enzymatic pathways in different species of animals and even in different strains of the same species. The various genetic factors which contribute to this heterogeneity in drug metabolism are presently being investigated under the rubric of pharmacogenetics. Another major factor affecting the metabolism of drugs is the age of the animal being tested. In some neonatal animals, the drug metabolizing enzymes are simply not functional until a certain period in maturation has been reached. Drugs that are administered prior to this period may as a result have prolonged and possibly toxic effects in the organism. Problems of this sort make up the area of developmental pharmacology. These genetic and ontogenetic variables are discussed at much greater length in Chapter 4.

Table 2.11 Activity of the Enzyme Alcohol Dehydrogenase in the Liver from Various Species[a]

Species	International Units/100 g Fresh Tissue
Man	200
Rhesus monkey	200
Horse	1540
Cow	110
Pig	320
Guinea pig	83
Rat	121
Mouse	115

[a] Data are from Moser et al. (1968).

Just as there may be competition between drugs for binding sites on plasma protein and cellular receptors, so too there may also be competition between drugs for the sites in the liver where the metabolizing enzymes are located. This competition is the basis for the treatment of alcoholism with the drug Antabuse (disulfiram). Normally, alcohol is converted by the body into acetaldehyde, which in turn is converted into acetic acid by the enzyme aldehyde dehydrogenase. Antabuse, however, competes with acetaldehyde for the metabolic activity of this enzyme with the result that the acetaldehyde metabolite of alcohol does not become transformed into acetic acid. As the amount of acetaldehyde in the blood increases, unpleasant physiological reactions such as nausea and vomiting begin to occur (cf. Hald and Jacobsen, 1948). The alcoholic who receives Antabuse on a regular basis supposedly is motivated to abstain from alcohol because of his anticipation of the unpleasant reactions he knows he will experience should he ingest any alcoholic beverages.

Besides affecting the metabolism of drugs by competition for metabolic enzymes, some compounds act directly on these enzymes to inhibit their activity. One such drug that is widely used in laboratory animals to impair drug metabolism is known by the commercial name of SKF 525A. Its potential effects on drug activity are evident whenever drug action is terminated by the liver. To illustrate, Axelrod et al. (1954) injected (i.p.) adult male rats with hexobarbital, a drug that induces a loss of the righting reflex. Half the animals also received an i.p. injection of SKF 525A approximately 40 minutes prior to receiving the hexobarbital. The animals in this latter group took approximately 80 minutes to recover their righting reflex compared with the control group, whose members recovered their righting reflex after only 27 minutes of hexobarbital treatment. Thus, by inhibiting the metabolism of hexobarbital, SKF 525A markedly increased the hypnotic actions of this drug. Additional information regarding drugs such as SKF 525A that inhibit liver microsomal activity may be found in Goldstein et al. (1969).

However, just as the activity of the drug metabolizing enzymes of the liver may be inhibited by compounds such as SKF 525A, a wide variety of drugs, all characterized by their relatively high lipophilia at physiological pH and their slow rates of biotransformation (Ciaccio, 1971), are able to stimulate the activity of these same enzymes. This stimulation may be manifest either by a direct increase in enzymatic activity, or by enzyme induction—an increase in the rate of synthesis of enzyme molecules, which is often accompanied by an increase in the density of the endoplasmic reticulum of the liver.

Stimulation of drug metabolizing activity generally leads to a more rapid inactivation of drugs with the result that blood peak levels are reduced and there is a more rapid rate of drug disappearance. Consequently, larger and larger doses may have to be administered to produce the original pharmacological or behavioral effect. This condition of decreased responsiveness to the effects of a drug resulting from prior exposure to it is termed tolerance. However, many of the microsomal enzymes lack substrate specificity and they will act upon a wide number of compounds. This can result in the related phenomenon of cross-tolerance, wherein tolerance to one drug confers tolerance to other drugs as well.

The phenomenon of tolerance is depicted in Fig. 2.6. In the experiment from which this figure is taken, pigeons were trained to peck a key for food reinforcement which was presented on the average of once every 3 minutes (VI 3'). Once a stable response rate had been established, the subjects were injected intramuscularly, intravenously, or orally with 10 mg/kg Δ^9-THC every other day, and were placed immediately after each injection into the experimental apparatus for the next 2 hours. It is quite evident from the figure that key-pecking behavior was clearly suppressed by the initial injections of the drug but that as the drug regimen was continued,

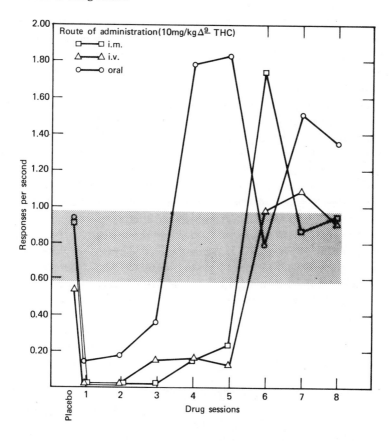

Fig. 2.6   Development of tolerance to Δ⁹-THC (10 mg/kg) in pigeons as a function of route of drug administration. The ordinate represents the mean number of responses emitted per second on a food rewarded key-pecking task. The abscissa represents drug sessions which occurred every other day. Nondrug sessions are not shown in the figure. The shaded area represents the range of high and low rates of responding for all birds for the mean of five sessions immediately prior to injection (from Abel et al., 1974).

key pecking returned to predrug control rates of responding. The mechanism underlying tolerance to this drug, however, has not been linked unequivocally to changes in liver drug metabolizing activity; at present the means by which tolerance to its effects develops is still unknown.

A number of additional points regarding the phenomenon of tolerance should be noted. The first is that tolerance to some drugs can occur very rapidly. For instance, tolerance to the hypothermic effects of Δ⁹-THC can be demonstrated clearly after a single injection in 15-day-old chickens

(Abel et al., 1972). With some drugs such as morphine, the tolerance conferred by a single dose of this drug can last for many months in the rat (Cochin and Kornetsky, 1964). This means that wherever there is a possibility of tolerance development, unless the experimenter is interested in the chronic effects of a drug per se, he should employ only drug-naive subjects. This is especially the case in determining dose-response relations between drugs and their effects, since tolerance development may distort or even completely obliterate the actions of some dosages of drugs.

A second point is that tolerance does not develop at the same rate for all the effects of a drug (cf. Abel et al., 1971a). Therefore, one should not pose questions such as "how fast does tolerance develop?," but rather, "how fast does tolerance to the X or Y effects of a drug develop?". For two very recent and thorough reviews of the literature dealing with these and other problems in the area of tolerance, the interested reader should consult Goldstein et al. (1969) and Kalant et al. (1971). Whatever the mechanisms underlying this phenomenon, tolerance itself emerges as a significant factor in the termination of drug activity and cannot be accounted for solely in terms of liver microsomal enzyme activity or increased rates of excretion.

Elimination

Drugs can be eliminated from the body by several routes. For instance, drugs such as alcohol and its metabolite acetaldehyde often are eliminated by expiration through the lungs. General anesthetics are eliminated also in this manner. Other drugs or their metabolites may be channeled through the bile duct into the gastrointestinal tract and if they are not reabsorbed back into the bloodstream, they are eliminated in the feces. However, the most common route for the elimination of drugs and/or their metabolites is via the kidney.

The functional unit of the kidney is the nephron, which is composed of a glomerulus and a tubule. The glomerulus acts as a filter which allows the passage of substances dissolved in the plasma to pass through it but blocks the passage of undissolved solutes such as those bound to plasma protein. The filtrate is then passed on to the tubule. The factors which govern reabsorption of materials from the tubule are identical to those which influence their movement across other cellular membranes. Drugs or metabolites that are still relatively un-ionized and lipid soluble diffuse readily across the tubule membrane back into the circulation; those that are ionized and are poorly lipid soluble do not pass back into the circulation and are excreted in the urine (see Fig. 2.7).

The physicochemical factors which affect the passage of drugs across cellular membranes in general can also be used to influence the excretion or retention of drugs at the level of the kidney. For instance, when a drug is in its un-ionized state, it will be more lipid soluble than when ionized, and therefore it will tend to diffuse back into the blood. Therefore an acidification of the urine (pH 4.5 to 8.5) will increase the ionization of slightly basic drugs, thus promoting their excretion; such procedures ought to have the opposite effect for acidic drugs.

The influence of urine pH on the elimination of amphetamine (pK_a 9.8) was demonstrated by Becket et al. (1965). These investigators administered d-amphetamine to human volunteers at three different times. Urine was collected at hourly intervals and the content of unchanged amphetamine was determined during each session. During the first session, no attempt was made to alter the pH of the urine. In subsequent sessions, the pH of the urine was either reduced to approximately pH 5.0 by the administration of ammonium chloride tablets or increased to approximately pH 8.0 by the administration of sodium bicarbonate. The effect of these alterations on the excretion of the drug was unequivocal. The low pH manipulation resulted in the excretion of 54.5% of the drug compared with

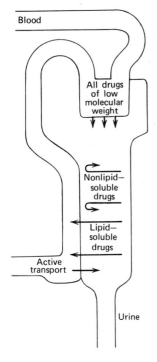

Fig. 2.7 Diagrammatic representation of excretion of drugs by the kidney (from Brodie, 1964a).

only 2.9% when the urine was made alkaline with sodium bicarbonate. Very similar findings have been reported by Astatoor et al. (1965).

The ability to affect the excretion of drugs in this manner can be very important from a therapeutic standpoint, since many problems of drug overdosage or drug poisoning can often be overcome simply by the physician's awareness of the physicochemical factors that affect the movement of drugs across cellular membranes.

DOSE-RESPONSE FUNCTIONS

The relationship between the dose of a drug and the response it elicits can be either graded or quantal. Graded functions are those in which the dependent variable may take on progressively increasing values as the dose is increased. A typical function that is often generated when the magnitude of response is plotted against drug dosage is that of a hyperbola. Such curves rise very steeply in the beginning and then flatten as dosage is increased continually (see Fig. 2.8, curve a).

Quantal relationships, on the other hand, are of the all-or-none variety. If the response occurs, it occurs maximally or not at all. The quantal dose-response curve thus gives rise to an entirely different kind of function since it represents the number of subjects at each dose that manifest a particular response (see Fig. 2.8, curves b and c).

In generating graded dose-response relationships, the magnitude of response at each of several doses is determined for a single biological system

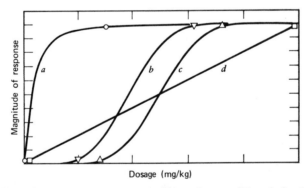

Dosage (mg/kg)

Fig. 2.8   Theoretical dose-response curves illustrating possible relationships between drugs and their effects. Curve a depicts a graded, increasing function. Curves b and c represent the all-or-none responses typical of biological variation. Curve d illustrates direct proportionality between dose and response (adapted from von Rossum and Ariens, 1962).

(see p. 90). The responsiveness of the individual can then be determined or else the investigator may take the mean response of several individuals at a particular dose in order to construct an average graded dose-response function.

To generate a quantal dose-response function, many more subjects must be used than is the case with the graded determination since the number of subjects responding or not responding to a given dose of drug is being determined. In toxicity studies, for instance, the questions often take the form of determining the number of deaths caused by ever-increasing doses of a given drug. The first requirement in answering such questions would be to obtain a large group of animals of the same species, age, sex, weight, etc., so that there would be a certain uniformity in the subject population. The animals would then be divided into groups and each would receive a different amount of drug. The number of subjects dying at each dose would then be recorded. If the data were then plotted in the form of a frequency polygon such as that depicted in Fig. 2.9, it would be readily apparent that not all of the subjects would die at the same dose: most of the subjects would die at the intermediate doses, and a few animals would die at the low and the high doses. Should a line be drawn connecting the middle of each of the bars, we would observe it to take the form of the bell-shaped curve typical of the normal frequency distribution commonly obtained whenever biological data are plotted in this way. This curve essentially reflects the fact that even though every attempt is made to minimize variability between subjects, biological differences will still remain despite the apparent homogeneity of the population from which the subjects are drawn. Such differences will become especially evident if the group of subjects being tested is relatively large.

Although drug data can be depicted readily by means of a frequency polygon such as that shown in Fig. 2.9, much more information typically is obtained when doses and responses are plotted in terms of a summation polygon, that is, when the proportion of subjects exhibiting a response is plotted versus drug dosage. When this is done, a sigmoid curve like that shown in Fig. 2.10 is invariably generated. This S-shaped curve is very similar to that obtained when graded dose-response relationships are examined. Despite these resemblances in shape, however, it should always be kept in mind that each function conveys a different type of information. The graded curve indicates how changes in the magnitude of response vary as the dose of a drug is increased or decreased. Quantal curves, on the other hand, indicate the frequency with which a given amount of drug induces a predetermined response. It is thus a reflection of the sensitivity of a given subject population to the effects of a particular drug.

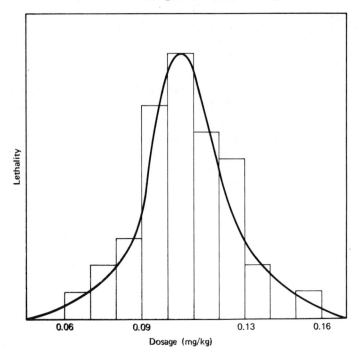

Fig. 2.9 Relationship between concentration of drug and frequency of death. Anesthetized cats were infused with ouabain and the amount of drug required to produce heart failure was determined. The dose in mg/kg was recorded and the number of animals dying at a particular dose were grouped together and plotted as shown in the graph. Most of the animals died in the dose range 0.09 to 0.13; however a few animals died after receiving much higher doses of the drug (modified from Marsh, 1951).

POTENCY

In plotting data in terms of dose-response functions, one soon becomes aware of the problem of choosing an appropriate dose from which to make comparisons between the effects of two or more drugs. For example, in Fig. 2.11, the curve for drug A is relatively steep compared with that for drug B. The variability associated with A is thus much greater than that associated with B. This means that small increases in the dosage of drug A will produce relatively large increases in whatever it is that is being measured. On the other hand, the slope of the curve for drug B is much flatter, and relatively large increases in the dosage of this drug will produce relatively small increases in the dependent variable. How then does one compare the effects of these two drugs? The answer is, it depends upon what one wishes to compare. Typically, drugs are compared in terms of their potency.

Drugs are said to be potent when they produce a large biological response at small dosages. In comparing the potency of two or more drugs, dose-response curves are first plotted and then the dosage of each drug that produces 50% of its maximal effect is determined. This is shown in Fig. 2.12 by the dotted lines, one of which projects horizontally from the ordinate at its median to the dose-response curve, the other of which drops vertically from the point on the curve where the intersection occurs relative to the abscissa. The point on the abscissa where the line falls is designated the "effective dose 50" and is written ED_{50}. If lethality were the dependent variable, this point on the abscissa would be designated the "lethal dose 50," written as LD_{50}. The drug with the lower ED_{50} or LD_{50} in terms of drug dosage, not magnitude of effect, would then be the most potent since

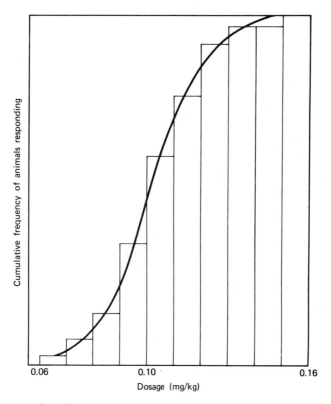

Fig. 2.10 Relationship between drug dose and response plotted as a summation polygon. A curve connecting the midpoints of each of the bars produces the sigmoid or "S" shaped curve shown in the figure (modified from Marsh, 1951).

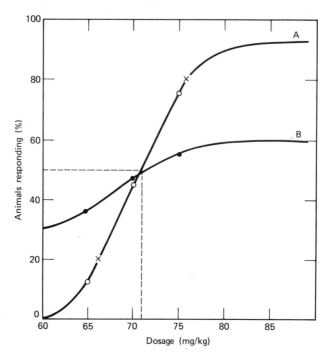

Fig. 2.11   Dose-response sigmoid curves of two hypothetical drugs with the same ED$_{50}$s but with different slopes.

the same intensity of response was elicited by less drug. Thus in Fig. 2.11, despite differences in variability between drug A and drug B, they are equipotent. Now consider Fig. 2.12. Here drug A produces the same intensity of response as B, but requires much less of a dose to do so. In this case, drug A is said to be more potent than drug B. Consequently, in comparing the dosage of two or more drugs required to produce a given magnitude of response at the same receptors, we are able to determine which of the two drugs is the more potent.

MULTIPLE DRUG EFFECTS

Very often a drug that is given for one purpose is found to produce other effects for which it was not intended if the dosage is increased. With anesthetic drugs, for instance, this second unwanted effect is sometimes death. Fig. 2.13 illustrates the fact that as the dosage of a hypothetical anesthetic drug is increased, two separate dose-response functions are generated, one for its anesthesia and one for its lethality. The fact that the two functions are parallel indicates that these two effects are being produced as a consequence of the actions of the drug on the same population of receptors. Death can also result from the actions of a drug on some mechanism entirely unrelated to the mechanisms by which it produced its intended effects. Should this in fact be the case, one would then not necessarily expect the dose-response curves to be parallel since a different population of receptors would be involved in each effect.

Given the fact that a drug may be toxic if too much of it is given, the dangers associated with its administration must be weighed against its desired effects. One measure of the safety of a given drug that is often cited is its therapeutic index (TI), which is defined as the ratio of the LD_{50} of a drug to its ED_{50}. For example, with an LD_{50} of 300 mg/kg and an ED_{50} of 100 mg/kg, the TI would be 3.0. This means that about three times as much drug would have to be given to produce death as would be needed to produce anesthesia in 50% of the subjects. Thus the higher the TI of a drug the less hazardous it is to life.

TIME COURSE OF DRUG ACTIVITY

Unless a drug is applied directly at its site of action, its activity will be characterized not only by the magnitude of its effects, but also by its latency of onset, its latency to peak effect, and its duration of action. The latency of onset refers to the time between the administration of the drug and the first observable indications that it is beginning to have some effect. Because a drug does not begin to exert any effects until its concentration

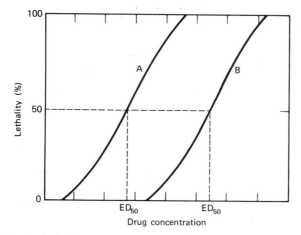

Fig. 2.12 Hypothetical dose-response curves. The horizontal distance between the two curves represents their relative potency. Drug A is relatively more potent than drug B since the same ED_{50} is produced with a lower concentration of drug.

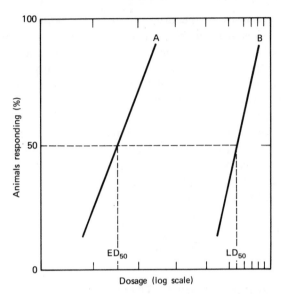

.Fig. 2.13 Hypothetical dose-response curves for the same anesthetic drug. Curve A represents the number of subjects experiencing anesthesia. Curve B represents the number of animals dying as the dosage is increased. The fact that the curves are parallel indicates that both effects are mediated by the same receptor mechanism (see text).

at its receptors is above threshold, the latency of onset will be determined by such bioavailability factors as the rate of absorption, distribution, etc. The latency to peak effect, on the other hand, refers to the time from the administration of the drug until its concentration at its site of action is maximal. This is determined not only by absorption and distributional factors but also by factors that inactivate the drug and carry it away from the area of its receptors, for example, metabolism and elimination. The third parameter, the duration of action, refers to the time from the onset of action until the drug no longer produces any observable effects. This phase is determined mainly by the rate of its metabolism and elimination. The time course of a drug's activity is thus influenced by the various pharmacodynamic factors which have been discussed at length throughout this chapter.

In determining the relationship between dose and response, it is obviously of importance to know the time course of action for a drug. If such information were not known, drug responses might be measured too soon or too long after drug administration. Since dose-response effects are expressed in terms of peak activity, it is apparent that one cannot compare the potency of two drugs if the effects of one of them are measured at its peak level and the effects of the other are measured at some point before or after peak activity. Thus in comparing certain parameters of drug action such as potency, familiarity with the time course of action of each drug is a prerequisite if that comparison is to be valid.

LOG DOSE-RESPONSE FUNCTIONS

In plotting the frequency distribution of the responsiveness of a population of subjects to a given drug, it is sometimes the case that the distribution is skewed when dosage is plotted on an arithmetic scale. In 1933, Gaddum showed that if drug dosage were plotted on a logarithmic scale instead of the usual arithmetic scale, dose-response data would take on the form of the normal frequency distribution; that is, the distribution of values would become symmetrical around the mean. Normalizing the distribution in this way meant that the data from biological studies could then be subjected to parametrical statistical tests such as the "t" test and the analysis of variance, without violating one of the basic prerequisites of these tests, namely, that the data being examined are distributed normally (cf. Edwards, 1965). Consequently, it is now almost customary in pharmacology to plot drug dosages logarithmically.

Another advantage of plotting dosages logarithmically is that various dose-response functions that might otherwise be difficult to compare become transformed into straight lines (see Fig. 2.14). Furthermore, by

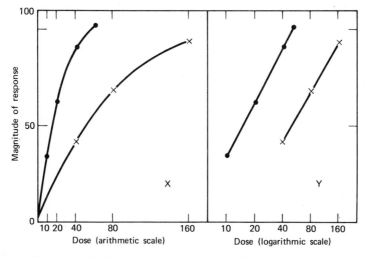

Fig. 2.14 Results of plotting drug dosage using an arithmetic scale (X) and using a logarithmic scale (Y) on the shape of the dose-response function (modified from Gaddum, 1959).

plotting drug dosage on a logarithmic scale, multiplicative differences between doses are changed into additive differences. For instance, intervals between doses that were previously double one another now become additive. As a result, it becomes possible to examine in more detail the initial phases of the dose-response curve which often tend to be very steep if drug dosage is plotted arithmetically. With a more detailed representation, investigators are then able to evaluate more closely the amount of change in response function that corresponds to small increases in drug dosage. This same advantage also relates to the terminal phases of the dose-response function where large doses of drug produce only very small increases in responsiveness. By plotting dosage logarithmically, those changes in responsiveness that were previously too small to depict on an arithmetical scale can now be shown in much greater detail.

3. Mechanisms of Drug Action

When pharmacologists speak of the mechanism of action of a drug, they are directing their comments to the wheres, the whys, and the hows of its activity. To the pharmacologist, it is simply not enough to describe the effects of a drug. He wishes to know why one drug produces a given effect and another does not. And he wants to know how that effect is produced. The answers to these questions are, of course, essential if pharmacology is ever to go beyond a cataloging of empirical drug effects to arrive at a statement of general principles of drug action. Although a complete explanation of drug action is not yet possible, pharmacologists have been able to generate a number of concepts which help to account for a great number of empirical observations. Foremost among these concepts is that of the drug receptor.

The fact that drugs act on some cells and not others, coupled with the observation that the biological activity of most drugs can be changed markedly by very minor alterations in their chemical structures, suggests that cells that are responsive to drugs contain reactive sites which are complementary in configuration to those of the drugs which act upon them. For lack of a better term, these sites have been termed receptors. It is assumed that whenever a drug and its receptors interact, certain physiological and biochemical changes occur at the site of action which act as a stimulus to produce a response. In pharmacology, drugs which initiate responses by interacting with these receptors are termed agonists, whereas compounds which prevent such interactions and which produce no responses of their own at the receptor are referred to as blocking agents or antagonists (anti-agonists).

Although the concept of the receptor constitutes a central tenet in pharmacology, no drug receptor has even been seen, even with the aid of the electron microscope. Instead, the actual existence of these cellular entities is very much a hypothetical inference, in the same way that the existence of pores in cellular membranes is a hypothetical inference. In both cases, these inferences are based upon certain facts that cannot be explained without presuming the presence of these structures somewhere in or on the cell itself. Although these receptors have not been isolated, many of them have been characterized on the basis of the reactivity of certain tissues to various agonists and antagonists. For instance, tissues that respond to acetylcholine are presumed to contain receptors resembling acetylcholine in configuration, whereas those which respond to norepinephrine are presumed to contain receptors similar in configuration to norepinephrine. In other words, drug receptors have generally been characterized on the basis of the compounds which react with them, rather than on the basis of direct observation of their appearance. The classification of receptors has thus been solely operational, the idea being that similarities and differences in the actions of various biologically active chemicals reflect similarities and differences in the receptors that mediate their activity (Furchgott, 1972).

However, stating that a drug acts on a particular receptor still falls far short of explaining what actually happens to the cell as a result of the drug-receptor interaction. In other words, the combination between a drug and its receptor does not itself constitute an explanation for the actions of that drug. Instead, it is really only the first step in a series of steps which eventually leads to a response.

In the case of the catecholamines, a number of experiments have now elucidated one of these next steps by showing that after an agonist of this type reacts with its receptor, a change in the cellular level of a substance known as cyclic AMP occurs. The idea has thus been proposed that cyclic AMP functions as a "second messenger' which goes on to do the work of the agonist inside the cell.

Cyclic AMP has been detected in a great many cells along with adenyl cyclase, the enzyme which catalyzes the formation of this substance from ATP. It has been shown that whenever adenyl cyclase activity is stimulated by a catecholamine, this stimulation can be antagonized by a β-adrenergic blocking agent such as propranolol (see Fig. 3.1), but not by any α-adrenergic blocking agents. Conversely, whenever adenyl cyclase activity is decreased by a catecholamine, this decrease can be antagonized by an α-adrenergic blocking compound such as phentolamine but not by any β-receptor blocking agents. These findings have suggested that the activity of adrenergic drugs at α and β-receptors is mediated by cyclic AMP, whose levels are either stimulated or inhibited by these agents, and that the receptors themselves may be integral parts of the adenyl cyclase systems in cells which contain α and β-receptors (Robinson et al., 1970).

Despite certain misgivings about the nature and the location of drug receptors, however, the notion of a specific reaction between a drug and

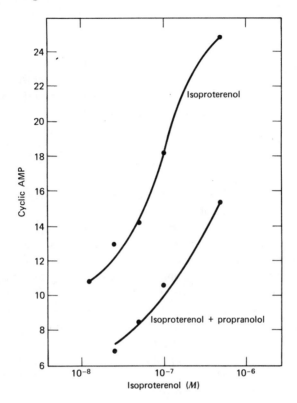

Fig. 3.1 Effects of isoproterenol and isoproterenol + propranolol on levels of cyclic AMP in rat uterus (from Robinson et al., 1970).

some specialized site in a cell is now generally accepted in pharmacology. Not only has it shown itself to be especially fruitful in accounting for many of the characteristics of drugs such as their specificity, but it has also offered a rationale for describing the actions of many drugs. Equally important, the concept of the receptor has stimulated a great deal of research directed at discovering the properties that make drugs agonists or antagonists.

It should not be concluded, however, that all drugs exert their effects via receptor mechanisms. Certain of the general anesthetics, for example, appear to depress cellular activity by temporarily altering the properties of cellular and subcellular membranes in a way that cannot be attributed to the molecular configuration of these drugs. This is a general effect that is shared by the sedative-hypnotic and other depressant drugs (see Chapter 5) and is referred to as structural nonspecificity. Details of the mechanism of action of these drugs are presented in the latter part of this chapter. It is to the characteristics of the receptor and the drug-receptor complex that we now turn.

THE RECEPTOR

The concept of the drug receptor goes back to Langley (1906), who on the basis of his studies with various drugs and their antagonists, hypothesized that there is a specific "receptive substance" in muscle tissue that serves as the site of action for various drugs such as nicotine and curare. This idea was developed subsequently by Ehrlich (1913), who postulated that all cells are characterized by "side chains," each with a different shape and chemical composition, and that only compounds with matching shapes and similar chemical compositions could affix themselves to these cellular "receptors" as he termed them. The next development in receptor theory was made by Clark (1937), who set the theory on a quantitative course by arguing that the biological effect produced by a given dose of active drug is directly proportional to the number of receptors occupied by that drug. The more intense the response, the more receptors occupied. When all the receptors are occupied, the effect produced by the drug is maximal.

At the same time that Clark and others were trying to develop the receptor theory into a general theory of drug action, other investigators were trying to discover where in the cell these hypothetical receptors might be located. A growing amount of evidence soon began pointing in the direction of the cell membrane. For example, one of the earliest experiments demonstrating that chemical receptors are located on or in cellular membranes was reported by Marsland (1934), who used the amoeba as his experimental preparation. Marsland found that when a drop of oil containing paraffin was brought into contact with the surface of an amoeba, the organism was rapidly narcotized and ceased to move. However, when droplets of this paraffin solution were injected directly into the interior of the amoeba, no narcosis resulted. Apparently, the narcotic effects of the paraffin on the amoeba arose from its action on the exterior of the organism's cell membrane rather than somewhere in the interior of the cell itself.

There is also a basic consideration which points to the location of drug receptors being in or on the cell membrane rather than in the interior of the cell. This consideration involves the fact that many substances such as acetylcholine and norepinephrine contain polarized groups, and therefore they do not readily diffuse through cellular membranes. However, they still have the potential for binding at the cell membrane surface and, once bound, for altering the properties of that membrane via their action on specific receptors (cf. Potter and Molinoff, 1972). In this respect, it is interesting to note that evidence for the reaction between serotonin and a specific kind of lipid, ganglioside, has been reported (Wooley and Gommi, 1964a, 1964b). Since lipids are involved in the structural and functional integrity of cellular membranes, this observation constitutes a further indi-

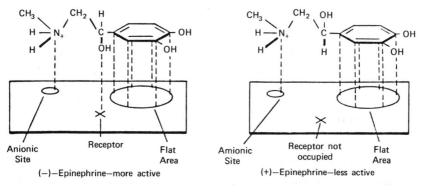

Fig. 3.2 Schematic diagram depicting the relationship between two isomers of epinephrine and their receptor. The figure indicates that (−)-epinephrine has a better "receptor fit" than (+)-epinephrine because each of its binding groups, the positively charged nitrogen, the alcoholic hydroxyl, and the aromatic ring, has a complementary receptor surface within which to fit. In the (+)-isomer, however, only two binding sites, the nitrogen and the aromatic ring, are able to occupy the receptor surface (from Daniels and Jorgenson, 1971).

cation that the receptors for the biogenic amines, at least, are located in the cellular membrane. For nerve cells, the postsynaptic receptors are believed to be coupled to a mechanism which can generate a change in the permeability of the cellular membrane, resulting in either a depolarization or hypopolarization of the neuron. However, because of the specificity of these receptors, if a molecular group is in a different position or is in an orientation different from that of the naturally occurring neurotransmitter, the response may not occur at all (see Fig. 3.2).

In addition, the enzymes associated with cellular activities have also been regarded for some time as one of the main receptor substrates upon which drugs may act in producing their effects, for example, the inhibition of acetylcholinesterase by physostigmine. Thus the ways in which structurally specific compounds affect the activity of enzymes associated with cellular functioning are yet another aspect of drug-receptor activity to be considered.

ANTAGONISM

When the biological effects of an agonist are either diminished or eliminated by another drug, this second compound is often referred to as a blocking agent or an antagonist. Actually, there are three different kinds of antagonism, only one of which can be termed pharmacological. The other two types involve chemical and physiological considerations; these will be discussed first.

Chemical Antagonism

This kind of antagonism occurs when the structure of the agonist is altered before it has a chance to act upon a receptor. For example, in cases of poisoning by heavy metal ions such as lead,* the chelating compound ethylenediaminetetraacetic acid (EDTA) is sometimes administered as an antidote because it binds lead ions to form a structure called a chelate complex, thereby rendering the harmful ion inactive.

Physiological Antagonism

A compound which produces an effect opposite to that of another compound is a physiological antagonist. This kind of antagonism involves each compound acting upon a distinct receptor site. For example, if norepinephrine were administered to an animal and its body temperature were lowered, norepinephrine could be considered to be an agonist. If this effect were subsequently reversed by the administration of serotonin, the latter could be regarded as a physiological antagonist. Conversely, if the order of administration of these compounds were reversed and serotonin increased body temperature and norepinephrine then lowered it, the norepinephrine would then be the physiological antagonist.

Pharmacological Antagonism

Only compounds that affect the reaction of agonists with their receptors can be designated pharmacological antagonists. This kind of antagonism is divided further into that which is competitive and that which is noncompetitive. Competitive antagonists combine with the same receptors as do agonists. In other words, they both possess affinity for the same receptor site. However, only agonists also possess intrinsic activity (see p. 107). Thus, whereas agonists precipitate some kind of response as a result of their receptor interaction, competitive antagonists do not, or at least they produce only a very weak response if they have some partial agonistic activity. Such antagonists are called "competitive" because their blocking effects may be overcome if the concentration of the agonist is increased. In such cases, the antagonism is said to have been surmounted. Overcoming the blockade of an antagonist is thus one of the tests that can be employed to determine whether an antagonist is of the competitive type.

* Poisoning by heavy metal ions occurs as a result of the combination of these ions with the free sulfhydryl ($-SH$) groups in enzymes. This has the effect of inhibiting their activity and because of their vital catalytic role, such inhibition eventually results in a cessation of cellular functioning.

In essence, competitive antagonists decrease the apparent affinity of agonists for their receptors (Goldstein et al., 1969). When dose-response curves are plotted for an agonist by itself and then for the same agonist in the presence of a competitive antagonist, the dose-response curve for the agonist is shifted to the right. However, neither the slope nor the maximum effect of the drug is altered.

Let us take as an example of the effects of a competitive antagonist, the blocking action of atropine on the otherwise stimulatory effects of acetylcholine on the guinea pig ileum.

Because it is rather difficult to study this reaction in the body itself, the ileum is removed and placed in a warm bath under conditions that will enable it to respond for long periods. By adding acetylcholine to the bath in which the ileum has been placed and by attaching to the ileum a device which can record its movements, it is possible to produce and record the same kinds of contracting responses that the tissue would normally have undergone if it were still in situ. Moreover, if the bath is soon replaced by a fresh medium not containing acetylcholine, the muscle begins to relax back to its original state. By systematically increasing the amounts of acetylcholine placed into the bath each time, it is possible to construct a dose-response function between the dose of acetylcholine and the magnitude of the contractions in the isolated guinea pig ileum.

It would then be possible to study the dose-response relationships between several other compounds and the contractions of the ileum, and on the basis of these results we could determine the potency of these compounds relative to acetylcholine (see p. 90). However, our objective is to study the effects of atropine in relation to acetylcholine. To do this, we repeat the dose-response testing of acetylcholine, but this time the bath medium in which the ileum is immersed contains a given amount of atropine sulfate. When this is done, we observe that acetylcholine is no longer able to make the muscle contract at the doses that were previously able to do so. However, if the doses of acetylcholine are increased, the muscle once more begins to contract and with the dose of acetylcholine increased still further, the muscle can be made to contract with an intensity equal to that observed before the atropine was present. If we wished, we could repeat the whole experiment and determine once again the dose-response function for acetylcholine in the presence of even more atropine sulfate in the bath water.

If we plot the log dose-response curves for acetylcholine by itself and acetylcholine in the presence of different doses of atropine, we would observe three curves similar to those in Fig. 3.3. The curve farthest to the left would be that for acetylcholine by itself. The one next to it would be that for acetylcholine in the presence of atropine, and the curve farthest to

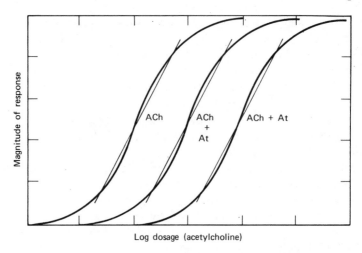

Fig. 3.3   Dose-response curves for acetylcholine (ACh) by itself and in the presence of increasing concentrations of atropine (At), a competitive antagonist. Note that the competitive antagonist causes the dose-response curve to be shifted to the right but does not affect the maximal response.

the right would be that for acetylcholine in the presence of even more atropine. The figure thus indicates that each new dose-response curve for acetylcholine in the presence of atropine is parallel to the control curve but is shifted to the right, making it appear as if acetylcholine had lost its potency. The more the concentration of atropine is increased, the farther to the right the curve is shifted and the "weaker" in potency acetylcholine is made to appear.

The explanation for this phenomenon is, as we have indicated previously, that atropine is a competitive antagonist. Whereas acetylcholine (the agonist) combines with the receptor and in so doing produces a response, atropine (the anti-agonist) combines with the same receptor but does not produce a response. Instead, it merely occupies a proportion of the total population of acetylcholine-sensitive receptors and makes them unavailable for occupancy by acetylcholine. However, as the dose of acetylcholine is increased, the agonist is able to displace the antagonist, atropine, from the receptors. In terms of the theory of drug action proposed by Ariens (1954) and Stephenson (1956), this means that whereas acetylcholine and atropine both possess affinity for the same receptor, only acetylcholine possesses intrinsic activity at this receptor.

Before leaving the topic of competitive pharmacological antagonism, we ought to mention some recent experiments involving the competitive opiate antagonist naloxone because of their great importance for the general topic of drug receptors. Using radioactively labeled naloxone, Pert and Snyder (1973) conducted some competition experiments between this drug and various opiate agonists such as morphine. First they placed different opiate drugs in a bath containing brain tissue from rats, mice, or guinea pigs, and then added radioactively labeled naloxone to the bath. The tissue was then dried and the amount of radioactivity in it was determined, the principle being that the greater the radioactivity, the greater the binding of the naloxone antagonist; the lesser the radioactivity, the greater the binding of the opiate agonists. With this biochemical method, Pert and Snyder found that the affinity for binding to nerve tissue correlated very highly with the pharmacological activity of the various opiates. In other words, naloxone was able to displace more of the weak opiates than the stronger opiates, weak and strong being defined in terms of their analgesic properties.

In a subsequent study, Pert et al. (1973) were able to demonstrate that by placing sodium chloride in the bath solution, they could selectively affect the binding of opiate agonists and antagonists. With sodium chloride present, agonists lost their ability to displace the naloxone antagonist that was already bound to nerve tissue. On the other hand, the presence of sodium chloride in the bath water was observed to increase the degree of binding for naloxone and other opiate antagonists very markedly.

In still another dramatic study, this same team (Kuhar et al., 1973) used this method to map the location of opiate receptors in monkey and human brain tissue. Their results showed that the opiate receptors were clustered mainly in the area of the limbic system. In the parts of the cerebral cortex where binding was observed, the greatest concentration occurred in the frontal lobes. The cerebellum and the brain stem had very little binding.

These findings thus represent the first direct demonstration of an affinity of an opiate drug for specific functional areas of the brain. Interestingly, these same areas are known to be involved in emotionality and analgesia, the main two motivational factors for which these drugs are used and abused.

In contrast to competitive antagonists, noncompetitive antagonists alter both the slope and the maximum effect of an agonist (see Fig. 3.4). This effect can occur via either the chemical or physiological mechanisms of antagonism that have already been outlined. Noncompetitive antagonism is reversible in many cases, however, as a result of the elimination of the compound from the body. Once the antagonist has been removed, the availability of the receptors it previously inactivated is restored, and maximal responsiveness to the agonistic effects of a given drug is once again possible. However, in the case of some compounds such as the insecticide parathion, the noncompetitive antagonism is irreversible.

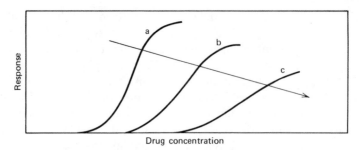

Fig. 3.4 Dose-response curves for an agonist (*a*) in the presence of increasing concentrations of a noncompetitive antagonist (*b* and *c*). Note that the noncompetitive antagonist causes the dose-response curve to be shifted to the right and also prevents the agonist from producing the same maximal response produced in its absence.

Parathion is an inhibitor of the enzyme cholinesterase, which destroys acetylcholine after it has been liberated from presynaptic endings. By interfering with the destruction of acetylcholine, parathion causes it to accumulate at postsynaptic receptors. This eventually results in paralysis of respiratory and circulatory centers, convulsions, and eventually death.

THEORIES OF DRUG ACTION

Occupation Theory

One of the earliest attempts to relate dose-response functions to drug receptor interactions was made by Clark (1937). In calculating the number of drug molecules necessary to elicit a pharmacological response, Clark concluded that only a relatively small proportion of the cell membrane could be involved in drug action. On this basis he proposed that drugs act at receptors and that the drug-receptor interaction could be formulated in terms of the law of mass action, following acceptance of the following assumptions: (1) the relationship between drugs and their receptors is rigid and analogous to that of a "lock and key" mechanism; (2) as a result, drugs, the chemical keys, elicit all-or-none responses in their receptors, the cellular locks. In other words, they open them or they do not open them. (3) The occupation of a particular receptor does not prevent other drugs from occupying other receptors; and (4) the magnitude of the elicited response is directly proportional to the number of receptors occupied by a drug.

Clark's basic premise that drug action is related to the number of "occupied" receptors is still generally endorsed by many investigators, although along with some of his other assumptions it has been subjected to modification. For example, the fact that some drugs produce very little effect of their own and yet are able to block the effects of other drugs suggested that they occupy receptors but still produce in them no response. This observation prompted Ariens (1954) and Stephenson (1956) to introduce the concepts of affinity and intrinsic activity, or efficacy as it is sometimes known, as characteristics of each drug. Affinity characterizes the degree of attraction of a drug for a receptor, regardless of whether or not it produces a response. Intrinsic activity, on the other hand, refers to the ability of a drug to produce an effect once the drug has combined with its receptors. This means that the higher the intrinsic activity of a drug, the fewer the number of receptors that have to be occupied to produce a given response. The assumption of intrinsic activity also challenges the assumption of an all-or-none receptor response, since it implies that the response of the receptor to a drug is one that is graded in nature, a characteristic shared by all known receptor mechanisms of the body. However, by means of some effect akin to spatial summation, the receptor responses sum up to become a generatorlike potential, resulting in an all-or-none cellular response. In the case of the nerve cell, this all-or-none response would be an action potential, the intrinsic activity of the drug stimulus being coded in terms of the frequency of impulse generation.

Drugs that possess both affinity and intrinsic activity are termed agonists; partial agonists are drugs that possess less affinity or less intrinsic activity than agonists. In general, drugs that produce parallel dose-response curves are assumed to be acting upon the same receptors, differing only in terms of their affinity. These drugs are able to produce the same magnitude of effect; that is, they possess equivalent intrinsic activity. Because of difference in affinity, however, it requires more of one than of another to do so.

Further evidence that the intensity of a biological effect does not depend solely on the number of receptors a drug occupies, as argued by Ariens and Stephenson, was introduced around the same time by Furchgott (1955) and by Nickerson (1956). These two investigators showed this to be the case by inactivating a proportion of the receptors in a given tissue preparation by treating them with a noncompetitive antagonist, after which they examined the dose-response functions produced by certain agonists. The rationale for these experiments was as follows: if the biological response to an agonist is directly proportional to the number of receptors it occupies, then the fewer receptors available, the lower ought to be (*a*) the magnitude of response and (*b*) the slope of the dose-response curve the agonist would be capable of producing. However, at low doses of the noncompetitive antagonist this did not occur. The maximal effect was not decreased nor was there any change in the slope of the dose-response function. It was only when relatively higher doses of the antagonist were given that the changes in maximal effect and slope occurred. These observations indicated that a maximal effect can be produced when only a proportion of the total number of available receptors is occupied by an agonist, suggesting that "spare receptors" or a "receptor reserve" exists above and beyond that necessary for the occurrence of a full biological response. The magnitude of a biological response to a drug would thus appear to be determined by the absolute number of receptors it occupies and by its own intrinsic activity. Consequently, even if a drug were to occupy only a few receptors, it could still produce a maximal biological response if it possesses relatively high intrinsic activity.

Rate Theory

As an alternative to the "occupation theory" of drug action, Paton (1961) has proposed what he has called a "rate theory." Paton's thesis is that the stimulant effect of certain drugs is proportional not to the number of receptors that are occupied, but rather to the rate of drug-receptor combinations; the faster the rate of association and dissociation of a drug with its receptors, the greater the number of impulses generated per unit time. In the case of agonists, there would be a high rate of association and dissociation between them and their receptors; in the case of antagonists, there would be a high rate of association, but a low rate of dissociation. In other words, many drugs are antagonists because they tend to remain in contact with receptors for a much longer time than do agonists. This means that the accessibility of agonists to their receptors is reduced.

In support of Paton's hypothesis, there is the observation that some antagonists elicit brief excitatory effects before their blocking actions occur. It is contended that this initial excitatory effect is the result of the initial association of the antagonist with the receptor. This would occur at a rapid rate since association would be near maximum during the initial phase of the drug-receptor interaction. Once a relatively sizable number of receptor sites became occupied, the rate of association would then fall below the level necessary for the elicitation of a biological response.

However, whereas rate theory is mostly supposition, occupation theory is known to be valid in the case of at least one kind of drug-receptor interaction, namely, that involving enzymes. On the other hand, it is possible that each theory may be applicable for different receptors, but at present neither theory is able to account for all the known facts surrounding the interaction between drugs and their receptors.

Macromolecular Perturbation Theory

In contrast to the occupation and rate theories, a number of proposals have been made which attempt to explain what actually happens when drugs and their receptors combine. These theories begin by challenging another of Clark's assumptions, namely, the idea of a rigid "lock and key" relationship between drugs and their receptors. Instead of being rigid, the receptor is regarded by some theorists as a structural component which changes its conformation in reacting with a drug. This "induced fit" hypothesis was proposed originally with respect to enzymatic activities (Koshland, 1959), but subsequently it has been extended to the drug-receptor interaction as well. For example, Belleau (1964) has proposed a "macromolecular perturbation" theory in which he argues that the interaction of a drug with a macromolecular protein receptor could have the effect of transforming that receptor molecule from its normal resting state into a conformationally active state, such that in the case of an agonist, the protein receptor becomes an active catalytic enzyme (specific perturbation). This enzyme would then affect the rate of certain activities already taking place in the cell. In the case of an antagonist, the drug would still transform the receptor from a resting to an active state, but the enzyme produced as a result of this transformation would not be catalytically active (nonspecific perturbation). A partial agonist would be a compound which produces a combination of both specific and nonspecific perturbations resulting in less overall active enzyme.

A somewhat related idea has been proposed by Nachmansohn (1959), who suggested that rather than producing an active enzyme, a compound such as acetylcholine might produce a conformational change in a receptor, which might then result in a structural alteration in the cell membrane resulting in changes in its ionic permeability. This in turn could cause a depolarization of the cell membrane or the generation of an action potential.

STRUCTURALLY NONSPECIFIC DRUGS

In contrast to those drugs whose biological activity is markedly affected by minor changes in their chemical structures, a wide variety of drugs such as the volatile general anesthetics, for example, ether, chloroform, nitrous oxide, and halothane, and the alcohols, for example, ethyl alcohol, all produce rather similar depressant effects on the CNS even though they possess widely disparate chemical structures. Since these compounds do not owe their pharmacological activity to their molecular configurations as much as to certain of their physical properties, they are often referred to as structurally nonspecific drugs. However, this distinction between compounds that are structurally specific versus nonspecific is often quite arbitrary since many drugs owe their biological effectiveness to a combination of both chemical and physical properties. This is especially the case when the biological activity of a drug arises as a consequence of both its overall chemical configuration, which enables it to form a complex with a receptor, and the physical properties of a particular functional group in the molecule, which are responsible for producing the pharmacological effect characteristic of the drug.

The dichotomy between structurally specific and nonspecific drugs thus should be seen as a conceptual rather than a factual distinction. To categorize one major class of drugs as structurally specific means that the major property by which its effects are produced is related primarily to its chemical configuration. This does not mean that it lacks physical properties by which its activity is also affected. These physical properties are still present; it is only that they do not appear to contribute as much to the total biological activity of the compound. The activity of structurally nonspecific drugs, on the other hand, is especially due to their physical properties. These compounds do not form complexes with receptors and for this reason it is difficult to account for their effects in terms of their chemical configurations.

At the turn of the century, it was believed that the effectiveness of these structurally nonspecific agents was related to their lipid solubility as measured by their partition coefficients between oil and water. As outlined in Chapter 2, these partition coefficients were obtained by placing a substance in a mixture containing equal volumes of lipid (e.g., olive oil) and water, and then determining the ratio of the concentration of each agent in the lipid phase relative to its concentration in the water phase (see Table 3.1). The observed relationship between depression or narcosis and the partition coefficient, noted simultaneously but independently by Overton (1901) and Meyer (1901) subsequently gave rise to the Meyer-Overton rule of anesthesia: "narcosis commences when any chemically indifferent substance has attained a certain molar concentration in the lipoids of the cell" (Meyer, 1937).

However, the Meyer-Overton law soon had to be modified when it was observed that many substances that were highly lipid soluble still had no narcotic properties. Moreover, the objection was raised also that the composition of the organic solvents such as olive oil which had been used in these partition experiments was not very comparable to the lipid material making up the cell membrane. The modification proposed by Ferguson (1939) was that rather than measuring the distribution of a substance in an oil-water mixture, a better way of estimating narcotic activity was to measure the concentration of a drug in the extracellular fluids. Since the

Table 3.1   Relative Solubility of Different Anesthetics in Water and Lipid[a]

Substance	Concentration in Water Phase (moles/liter)	Concentration in Lipid Phase (moles/liter)	Partition Coefficient (Lipid/Water)
Ethyl alcohol	0.33	0.033	0.10
n-Propanol	0.11	0.038	0.35
Antipyrine	0.07	0.021	0.30
Barbital	0.03	0.041	1.38
Phenobarbital	0.008	0.048	5.9
Thymol	0.000047	0.041	950

[a] Data are from Meyer and Hemmi (1935).

amount of drug present in this phase would be equal to the amount of drug in the biophase, that is, the biologically active phase of the cell, the drug's thermodynamic or chemical potential could be determined. Ferguson found that this chemical potential did indeed closely reflect the narcotic activity of a drug. This finding suggested that the important factor in narcosis was the extent of a drug's saturation in the biophase of a membrane and led to Ferguson's law: "substances which are present at the same proportional saturation in a given medium will have the same degree of biological action."

Since nerve tissue is largely made up of lipid material, it is not surprising that the central nervous system is the main site of action of these lipophilic drugs. Apparently, the narcotic action of these agents arises as a result of their effects on the neuronal membrane itself rather than the interior of nerve cells since, as noted earlier in this chapter, these compounds act as depressants when applied to the exterior of a cell but not when they are placed directly inside the cell (e.g., Marsland, 1924). In a more recent series of experiments, Narahashi and his co-workers (Narahashi et al., 1967, 1970; Frazier et al., 1970) have also shown that the action potentials in perfused axons from which all the axoplasm has been removed are blocked by anesthetic drugs, and that these effects also can be produced using quaternary forms of those anesthetic compounds which are characterized by their inability to penetrate membranes very readily. Furthermore, although the action potential is blocked, the resting potential of the nerve cell remains relatively unaffected by the bulk accumulation of these drugs in the lipoprotein cell membrane. This suggests that the effect of these drugs probably is accomplished through an interference with those properties of the cell membrane which change during a depolarization, for example, a widening of the cell membrane pores. The end result of this "stabilization" of the nerve cell membrane (cf. Shanes, 1958) is a general depression of nerve activity.

SELECTIVITY AND SPECIFICITY OF DRUG ACTION

If a population of receptors has a high degree of specificity, only a few drugs will possess the structural and/or physicochemical features that will permit a drug-receptor combination. However, even though receptors may be highly selective in character, they may be located at more than a single anatomical site. For example, the receptors for many of the neurotransmitters such as acetylcholine and norepinephrine are distributed throughout the body, so that drugs that act on these receptors in the CNS activate these same receptors in other parts of the body as well, producing thereby so-called "side effects." The problem thus arises as to how to account for the relatively high specificity of action of many of the drugs that act primarily on the central nervous system. One answer to this problem takes a cue from the study of the bioavailability factors which affect the movement of drugs in general. For instance, if the blood-brain barrier were slightly different in structure or physicochemical properties in various anatomical regions of the brain, making it selectively permeable to drugs with slightly different physicochemical properties, then the specificity of action of many drugs could be accounted for on the basis of their localized distribution into different areas of the CNS (cf. Seeman, 1972).

TOLERANCE

One of the most intriguing problems associated with drug action is the manner by which the body adapts to the effects of some drugs. This adaptation in responsiveness to the actions of a drug as a result of prior exposure to it is termed drug tolerance and has been already introduced as one of the ways by which drug activity is terminated in the body. However, tolerance is a phenomenon that is also fundamental to considerations of drug dependence (see below) and of drug mechanisms in general. Therefore, this phenomenon is now examined in detail.

The chief characteristic of drug tolerance is that it is necessary to administer an increase in the amount of drug to produce the same magnitude of effect as that observed following its initial administration. If tolerance develops following a single administration of drug or after a few doses administered over a brief period of time, it is called "acute" tolerance or "tachyphylaxis." On the other hand, if tolerance takes place over an extended series of administrations, it is referred to as "chronic" tolerance. However, the distinction is highly subjective and is meaningless in certain situations. For example, with chronic daily administrations of Δ^9-tetrahydrocannabinol to young chicks, complete tolerance to the hypothermic effects of this drug requires approximately 14 injections if the daily dosage is 10 mg/kg. However, if the first dose is 180 mg/kg and the second is 10 mg/kg, then the same degree of tolerance as was seen in the case of the former drug regimen is evident by the second injection (Abel et al., 1972). This observation implies that the distinction between what is called "acute" and what is called "chronic" tolerance may be more a result of the dosage schedules used by various experimenters than a result of any differences in the rate of tolerance development by specific tissues (Hug, 1972).

There are certain additional characteristics associated with the phenomenon of tolerance which should be noted. For instance, the rate and extent of tolerance development have also been found to vary with the response being measured, the animal species being tested, the drug being investigated, and the time between successive administrations (see Seevers and Deneau, 1963). Furthermore, tolerance may not develop to all the pharmacological effects of a given drug. For example, tolerance has been observed for many of the effects of morphine, but not for the miosis (pinpoint pupil) and constipation associated with its usage. This implies that tolerance does not involve some fundamental change in the organism but rather some specific functional alteration either in a particular organ, group of tissues, or receptors. Quite possibly more than one mechanism may be involved in the phenomenon of tolerance (Kalant et al., 1972).

Currently, the only proposed mechanism for drug tolerance for which there is much support involves an increase in the liver microsomal enzymes which metabolize certain classes of drugs such as the sedative-hypnotics (e.g., ethyl alcohol, the barbiturates, and minor tranquilizers). This tolerance is manifested by a shortening of the duration of action of these drugs. Since these enzymes are not very specific in their activity, they sometimes act to shorten the duration of activity of other drugs as well. This lack of specificity is thus able to account for the phenomenon of "cross-tolerance," which refers to a decreased responsiveness to one drug as a result of prior exposure to another drug. In general, however, cross-tolerance typically develops to drugs that produce similar pharmacological effects.

Although part of the tolerance observed with many drugs can be traced to an induction of the liver microsomal enzyme systems which are responsible for their metabolism, this cannot account for the development of tolerance to drugs which are administered intracerebrally or intraventricularly (e.g., Tilson and Sparber, 1971; Watanabe, 1971) or to drugs such as barbital which undergo very little metabolism. Moreover, Kalant et al. (1971) point out that the main result of an increase in metabolic activity is a shortening of the duration of activity of a drug. This would have only a very negligible effect on the intensity of pharmacological effects if drugs are administered parenterally, however, because their onset of activity is usually much too rapid to be affected by the slow rate of metabolic inactivation (see also Goldstein et al., 1968, pp. 559).

At the level of hypothetical mechanisms of tolerance there are those theories that propose (*a*) differential rates of absorption, distribution, and/ or excretion between tolerant and nontolerant animals; (*b*) a decreased access of drugs to their sites of action; (*c*) a cellular adaptation at some physiological level; and (*d*) an occupation and saturation of receptor sites which prevent subsequent access of the drug to these sites.

Some of these hypotheses are more probable than others. The mechanism suggested in (*a*) is quite unlikely since alterations of this sort should influence all drugs to the same extent. This means that the tolerance exhibited to one drug should be conferred upon all drugs administered by the same route. This is clearly not the case. Secondly, if a diminished rate of absorption or distribution were involved, then no evidence of tolerance should occur if a drug were administered intravenously. However, tolerance does occur when drugs are administered by this route. In the case of differential distribution, it is conceivable that an increased binding to plasma protein could result in a decreased concentration of the drug in the blood. This would involve a substantial increase in the protein fraction of the blood, however, and little evidence is presently available in support of this proposal (cf. Hug, 1972). Alternatively, one could envision a lasting change in the pH of the urine of tolerant animals, but this pH change should affect the rate of excretion of other drugs as well. However, at present there is no evidence in support of this sort of mechanism either (Hug, 1972).

The evidence for the second hypothesis, namely, a decreased access to the site of action, is also largely negative. In studies which have directly measured the concentration of drug in the brain of tolerant versus nontolerant animals, meaningful differences have not been found. Studies using radioactively labeled compounds to trace the amounts of compound at various sites in the bodies of tolerant and nontolerant animals have likewise not been encouraging (see Kalant et al., 1972).

Arguments for an altered cellular responsiveness to drugs as a result of tolerance have been entertained for quite some time. In recent years, these arguments have been formulated in light of immunological concepts which postulate the formation of antibodies following the administration of antigens (=drugs) into the body. Although some investigators (e.g., Cochin, 1972) feel there is merit in this analogy, there is little in the way of well-documented evidence to support this supposition.

The remaining hypothesis proposes that a drug may reduce either the number or the rate of drug-receptor interactions for subsequent administrations of the same or related drugs, by forming a long-lasting complex with its receptors. This implies that the drug antagonizes its own subsequent effects by making access to receptor sites unavailable. Although there is evidence that some drugs do act as "self-antagonists" (cf. Rang and Ritter,

1969), this kind of mechanism seems unlikely in view of the fact that tolerance sometimes lasts as long as a year with drugs such as morphine; this would mean that drug receptors would be occupied for an extraordinarily long time, a possibility that is conceivable but difficult to accept (cf. Cochin, 1972).

Alternatively, tolerance could arise as a result of an increase in the total number of active receptors (Collier, 1966). This hypothesis has been formulated in light of the demonstrations of induced enzyme activity which were described above. An increase in the number of receptors would mean that a greater number of them would have to be affected by a drug for it to produce an effect. Although this hypothesis is also conceivable, before it can be realistically entertained, it would seem that some better understanding of receptor mechanisms in general is needed. Finally, there is one version of receptor theory (Furchgott, 1956) which postulates that maximal drug responses occur when an agonist occupies only a small proportion of the total number of available receptors. This implies that there are a great many "spare receptors" that remain unoccupied during the activity of a drug. An increase in the number of additional drug receptors would therefore be of no significance if this hypothesis were to be proved.

A number of formulations relating to potential mechanisms for drug tolerance have now been outlined. Unfortunately, none of them provides an unequivocal account of the empirical data. However, these hypotheses do incorporate many of the concepts and principles representative of pharmacology in general, and for this reason alone they are worthy of consideration. As more information regarding pharmacological principles becomes available, it is almost certain that a satisfactory explanation for the phenomenon of tolerance will be forthcoming.

PHYSICAL DEPENDENCE

In addition to tolerance, the repeated use of some drugs may also induce a state of drug dependence which is defined as a "compulsive" pattern of drug-seeking behavior. This definition recognizes two different kinds of drug dependence—that which is physiological and that which is psychological in origin.

Seevers and Deneau (1963) characterize physiological dependence as a "state of latent hyperexcitability which develops in the cells of the central nervous system of higher animals following frequent and prolonged administration of the morphine-like analgesics, alcohol, barbiturates and other depressants." This state is manifested as an abstinence syndrome upon abrupt termination of drug administration (or in the case of the morphine-like analgesics, upon administration of specific narcotic antagonists). The compulsive drug-seeking behavior associated with dependence of this type is sometimes referred to as "addiction."

Psychological dependence refers to the continuing use of drugs in order to maintain a subjectively acceptable state of well-being. Abrupt termination of drugs to which a psychological dependence has formed generally produces an unpleasant sensation, but there is no possibility of confusing these sensations with those manifested in the abstinence syndrome. The parallel to addiction in the case of psychological dependence is "habituation." This term refers to a continuing use of drugs which are considered to have no serious or harmful effect to either the individual or society, although the emphasis is on the latter. For example, the use of tobacco can have harmful effects on the individual. However, continued use of this substance is not likely to affect others. Differences between psychological and physical dependence are summarized in Table 3.2.

Table 3.2   Characteristics of Psychological and Physical Dependence

Psychological Dependence	Physical Dependence
1. Desire (but no compulsion) for continued use of drug	Compulsion to continue use of drug
2. Little tendency to increase dose (minimal tolerance)	Marked tendency to increase dose (tolerance)
3. No major physical symptoms upon withdrawal	Major physical symptoms upon withdrawal
4. Adverse effects restricted mainly to individual	Adverse effects to both individual and society

Although the initiation of drug-taking behavior has been attributed to sources such as pain or anxiety reduction and euphoria, the avoidance of the abstinence syndrome appears to be motivation enough for the maintenance or continued drug usage. This etiological pattern has been demonstrated clearly in the laboratory with animal subjects. The procedure is basically that of training the subject to make some kind of operant response such as lever pressing to obtain food, water, etc., and then training it to press some other manipulandum to activate an injection pump which delivers a predetermined amount of drug intravenously through an indwelling cannula. With this procedure it is possible to investigate the reinforcing value of various drugs along with their potential for "drug abuse" (see Fig. 3.5).

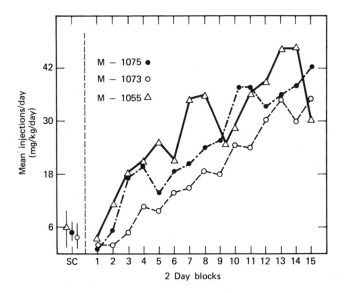

Fig. 3.5 Lever-pressing frequency for saline (averages and range) for 7 days, and for morphine reinforcement (1.0 mg/kg) for 30 days (2-day averages). During the predrug sessions, each lever press resulted in the infusion of saline for three monkeys. During the next 30 days, lever presses resulted in the infusion of morphine; the figure shows that saline infusion had little effect on the frequency of lever pressing. In contrast, the infusion of morphine following lever pressing resulted in an increased rate of responding, thus demonstrating that morphine acts as a "reinforcer" for this kind of behavior (from Schuster, 1970).

Under conditions such as these, some animals develop dependence to nearly every drug found to possess drug dependence liability in man (Schuster and Thompson, 1969). More importantly, this kind of approach has placed the phenomenon of drug dependence in an experimental framework. Besides giving added insight to clinical impressions of drug abuse, it has also enabled investigators to explore some of the genetic and environmental variables which influence initial drug administration, rates of self-administration, rates of development of drug dependence, and the relative reinforcing value of different compounds (see review by Schuster and Thompson, 1969). In summary, studies of this sort demonstrate that drugs possess direct positive reinforcement properties which can serve as the motivation for initiating drug-taking behavior. Should the subject become dependent, continued drug administration can be understood as being motivated by avoidance of the physical discomfort associated with abstinence.

This approach, however, only provides a behavioral context in which drug-taking behavior can be understood. It does not elucidate the mechanisms underlying the phenomenon of drug dependence nor does it explain why drug dependence occurs to some drugs and not others, or why the abrupt termination of some drugs precipitates an abstinence syndrome.

There are two characteristics of drug dependence which must enter into any consideration of the mechanism(s) responsible for this phenomenon. The first is that physical dependence always is accompanied by tolerance (although tolerance need not be associated with dependence). This invariability has prompted Collier's (1966) observation that physical dependence is the price that the body pays in adapting itself to the effects of many drugs. The second characteristic of physical drug dependence is that withdrawal of a drug to which a dependence has been formed, or treatment with an antagonist, will produce effects that are directly opposite to those observed with chronic administration of the drug. For example, morphine produces a general depression of nerve cells in the CNS. Abrupt termination of morphine, or treatment with a narcotic antagonist such as nalorphine, however, induces a marked hyperexcitability in the same cells that were initially depressed and a general inhibition of ongoing behavior (see Fig. 3.6).

To date, all the theorizing that has been directed at explaining this phenomenon has been formulated around the principle of homeostasis. The notion that all the vital mechanisms of the body have as their sole object the preservation of a relatively constant "milieu interieur" is one that has its origins in hoary antiquity. The term homeostasis, however, was coined only in this century (Canon, 1932). Briefly, it refers to the self-regulating aspect of the bodily mechanisms in which "any tendency towards change is automatically met by increased effectiveness of the factor or factors which resist the change" (Canon, 1932). As applied to physical dependence, the homeostatic compensation that occurs as a result of tolerance is assumed to continue in the absence of the drug and to produce a physiological reaction of its own which is no longer counteracted by the pharmacological effects of the drug. The net result is the increased excitability observed as an abstinence syndrome. The following hypotheses are essentially elaborations of this formulation.

In the "pharmacological redundancy" hypothesis outlined by Martin (1968), activity in the CNS is considered to be mediated by parallel pathways which are differentially sensitive to the effects of drugs. When the primary pathways become inactivated by certain compounds, the "redundant" neural circuits assume a much greater role in the transmission of neural impulses in the CNS. Evidence for the existence of such "redundant pathways" has been presented by Martin (1970; Martin and Eades, 1967) and is supported by the fact that upon destruction of certain areas of the brain, other areas appear to take over the functions previously subserved by the destroyed tissue. The occurrence of tolerance thus would be accounted for in this hypothesis by a greater efficiency in those redundant pathways which subserve the functions previously mediated by the primary pathways. Termination of drug administration, however, would remove the selective blockade in the primary pathways and as they became operational once more, the target tissues now innervated by both the primary pathways and the redundant pathways would become overstimulated, thus accounting for the hyperexcitability of the abstinence syndrome.

This theory is, of course, quite similar to that described in connection with Collier (1966). For example, by substituting the idea of "silent receptors" for "redundant pathways," we have pretty much the same formulation. Thus, as the activity of those receptors which react to endogenous excitatory neurotransmitters becomes inhibited by a drug, "silent receptors" are either induced or rendered functional. This increase in the number of active receptors accounts for tolerance. After removal of the drug from the previously blocked receptors, the total number of active receptors is in-

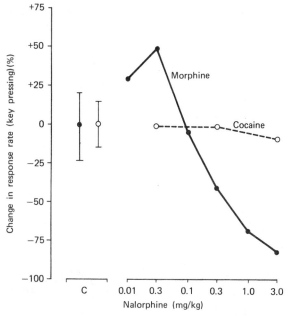

Fig. 3.6 Effects of the narcotic antagonist nalorphine on rate of key pressing rewarded by either morphine or cocaine injections. Monkeys first were trained to press a key in order to receive injections of these drugs. Animals then received saline (C) followed by nalorphine. Pretreatment with this antagonist had no effect on responding for cocaine reward but did inhibit morphine-reinforced behavior, at doses of 0.3 mg/kg and greater (modified from Goldberg et al., 1972).

creased suddenly and a marked hyperexcitability of those tissues containing these receptors is the result.

The theories of Shuster (1961) and Goldstein and Goldstein (1961) can be seen in a similar light. Both theories propose that certain drugs inhibit the production of neurotransmitters and that this results in a depression of neural activity. Continued drug administration, however, results in an increased activity of the enzymes that synthesize these transmitters, thereby compensating for the initial inhibitory activity of the drug (tolerance). Drug withdrawal terminates the inhibitory effect on transmitter production and together with the increased levels produced by enzymatic activity, there is an excess of transmitter present in the area of the synapse which manifests itself in postsynaptic hyperexcitability. A summary of the evidence in relation to neurotransmitters and both tolerance and physical dependence can be found in Smith (1972) and Wikler (1972).

The "pharmacological denervation supersensitivity" hypothesis proposed by Jaffe and Sharpless (1968) represents the converse to the hypotheses of Shuster (1961) and Goldstein and Goldstein (1961). Instead of an increase in neurotransmitter production, the basic premise of this hypothesis is that the latent hyperexcitability associated with the abstinence syndrome is due to the occurrence of "disuse supersensitivity" analogous to the "denervation supersensitivity" that develops in peripheral tissues that have been surgically or pharmacologically deprived of normal nervous input. In other words, the hypothesis proposes an increase in the sensitivity to neurotransmitter substances in those tissues which have been deprived of their normal nervous input because of some inhibitory activity of certain drugs. If these drugs are then withdrawn, the input to these tissues is restored and the supersensitized tissue responds with hyperexcitability. Although this hypothesis originally was based on observations of such hyperexcitability at peripheral sites, similar effects have been demonstrated recently for those central mechanisms which regulate body temperature (Friedman et al., 1969).

Although each of these hypotheses is plausible, it is not possible at this time to pass final judgment upon them because the specific neural pathways, receptors, neurotransmitters, enzymes, target tissues, that drugs act upon have not been identified to sufficient extent to permit direct experimental verification. Until such time as these studies can be conducted, those changes which occur during tolerance and dependence can be regarded only as correlates of these phenomena (Kalant et al., 1971).

Recently, however, a new insight into the possible mechanisms underlying physical dependence has been reported by Kerr and Pozuelo (1971) which implicates the hypothalamus in both the development of tolerance and physical dependence to morphine. The role of the hypothalamus in physical dependence was suggested several years ago by Andrews (1943) on the basis of electroencephalographic records from various areas of the brain that were recorded during drug withdrawal. Additional evidence has been reported by Lomax and Kirkpatrick (1967). The methodology used by Kerr and Pozuelo (1971) to investigate the role of the hypothalamus in physical dependence was basically that of lesioning various areas of this structure and observing the effects of these lesions on the development of tolerance and abstinence. This approach revealed that lesions in the ventro-medial area of the rat hypothalamus not only reversed morphine tolerance but also abolished the withdrawal syndrome, suggesting that this area may be either a main neural center or else one of the important relay sites in the mechanisms of tolerance and physical dependence. Lesions in the immediate vicinity of the ventromedial hypothalamus did not affect the dependence syndrome nor did lesions in the lateral hypothalamus or medial forebrain bundle, although lesions in the septal nuclei did have some atten-uating effects. Although these investigators did not explore the effect of cortical lesions on dependence, ti has been reported previously that absti-nence syndromes can be induced in decorticated dogs and decerebellated dogs (Essig, 1962, 1964; Wikler, 1950). This suggests that the physical site of dependence may be the result of the actions of certain drugs on quite limited nuclear areas in the central nervous system (Kerr and Pozuelo, 1971).

4. Sources of Varibility in Drug Activity

Even in situations where behavior is brought under the influence of rigorous stimulus control, individual differences in the response to drugs emerge. Although the number of parameters affecting drug activity is virtually limitless, there are certain variables associated with the actions of drugs which warrant special attention. These variables are the subject matter of this chapter.

GENETIC FACTORS

Since the various phyla of animal species differ from one another along numerous dimensions, it is not surprising that the response to drugs by different species may vary not only in quantitative terms, but may be qualitatively at variance as well. The response to morphine is the classic example for illustrating such interspecies differences since this drug has an excitatory effect in horses, donkeys, cattle, sheep, pigs, goats, cats, and mice, but has a depressant action in dogs, rabbits, rats, guinea pigs, and birds. Even within strains of the same species, differences in drug action may emerge. For example, social aggregation markedly increases the toxicity of amphetamine in Swiss-Webster, but not in DBF_1 or DBA/2 mice (Weaver and Kerley, 1962). Interspecies and strain differences such as these compound the problems that the pharmacologist faces in searching for the mechanism of action of drugs and also limit the generalities that can be drawn from any particular experiment.

On the other hand, although differences in the response to drugs between and within species may present an obstacle to some kinds of problems these same differences can provide valuable leads for investigating the genetic determinants of drug action. As a corollary, differences in the response to drugs may point out the source of genetic differences between animals (Meier, 1963). By simultaneously evaluating drug effects in two or more selected species or strains of animals, it may be possible to identify genotypic factors which contribute to a particular drug effect, and from that to gain insight into the basis for individual variability in drug action.

Since certain drug effects are presumed to depend upon drug-receptor interactions, interspecies differences in drug responsiveness may be due either to qualitative differences in receptor structure, distribution, sensitivity, etc., or to pharmacodynamic variables which affect the access of drugs to their receptor sites. An indication that there are inherited differences in receptor activity may be inferred from the now classic study by Fox (1932), in which he discovered that only certain humans are able to detect the taste of phenylthiourea. Either the receptors that are necessary for the detection of phenylthiourea are not present in many humans, or else they are present but are nonfunctional. It is thus evident that not only must one be cautious in extrapolating experimental results from animals to man, but even when the subject population is human, a certain amount of prudence must be exercised in generalizing drug responsiveness from one individual to the next.

The study of genetic influences on drug action, termed pharmacogenetics, has recently been the focus of considerable interest in pharmacology. Comprehensive reviews of this literature may be found in Fox (1967), Jacob (1971), Kalow (1962), Meier (1963), LaDu (1971), and Steinberg and Sheba (1968); only a few of the more interesting of these are reported here.

One of the most widely cited experiments in the field of pharmacogenetics was conducted by Quinn et al. (1958). These investigators administered a sedative-hypnotic drug, hexobarbital, to mice, rabbits, rats, and dogs, and measured the hypnotic effect of the drug in these various species simply by observing the duration of their loss of righting reflex ("sleeping time"). Whereas mice "slept" for an average of 12 minutes, rats slept for about 90 minutes following administration of the same dose of hexobarbital (100 mg/kg) by the same route (i.v.). With the mouse as a reference point, the relative duration of "sleeping time" for the mice, rabbits, rats, and dogs was 1:4:8:26, respectively. These differences were found to be correlated positively with the plasma half-life of the drug in each species and inversely with the rate of metabolism of hexobarbital by the hepatic microsomal enzymes in each species. Thus the differences in "sleeping time" apparently were related to interspecies differences in enzymatic activity.

Species differences in drug metabolism are another especially important consideration in pharmacogenetics. Because of qualitative differences in the metabolic pathways by which drugs are inactivated, or quantitative dif-

ferences in the metabolic enzymes common to a number of species, the
same dose of drug may produce a particular reaction in one species that
does not appear in another (cf. Williams, 1971). This is especially apparent in circumstances wherein a metabolite rather than the parent compound is the active agent.

An interesting example of the influence of genetic differences in response
to drugs comes from a study by Burns and co-workers (1955). In testing
the addictive potential of the narcotic analgesic, meperidine, Burns failed
to observe either physical dependence or tolerance to this compound in
dogs. Direct implementation of meperidine as a therapeutic agent in man
on the basis of this observation would have been imprudent, however, since
meperidine has just the opposite effect in humans. The reason for this dis-
parity is that in the dog, this drug tends to be inactivated and eliminated
so rapidly that it does not remain in the bloodstream long enough for tolerance or dependence to develop (Brodie and Reid, 1971). In man, the
metabolism and elimination of meperidine is less rapid with the result that
both tolerance and physical dependence occur (see Table 4.1).

Table 4.1   Metabolic Inactivation of Drugs in Man, Monkey, and Dog[a]

	Half-Life (hours)		
Species	Meperidine	Antipyrine	Phenylbutazone
Man	5.5	12	72
Monkey (Rhesus)	1.2	1.8	8
Dog	0.9	1.7	6

[a] Modified from Burns (1968).

One of the problems that arises in comparing drug effects in different
species is the specification of an acceptable base line from which to make
valid comparisons. Because of morphological and physiological differences,
comparative studies of drug action can result in extremely problematical
inferences. One pathway through the genetic maze that has been advocated
is that of using the plasma levels of free drug in each species as the standard referent with which to compare the effects of the drug (Brodie and
Reid, 1971). For instance, to obtain a plasma concentration of 3 μg/liter
for some drugs requires administration of 200 mg/kg of that drug if the
subject is a rabbit, compared with only 1 mg/kg if the subject is a human
(Koppanyi and Avery, 1966). The effective dose thus is not the administered dose, but the amount of drug in the blood (assuming that this reflects the effective concentration of drug at its site of action).

Brodie and Reid (1971) contend that dosages of drugs, when expressed in terms of milligrams per kilogram body weight, bear little relationship to the actual blood levels of a drug in different species of animals because each species differs not only in terms of the kinds of enzyme systems it possesses, but also in terms of the mechanisms for the absorption of drugs into the bloodstream, the binding of drugs to plasma proteins, kidney excretion, etc. When comparisons are made on the basis of equal plasma levels of free drugs, however, the levels of responsiveness of the various species tend to become more similar to each other than when comparisons are made on a usual milligram per kilogram basis (Brodie and Reid, 1971; cf. Koppanyi and Avery, 1966).

On the other hand, one must not lose sight of the possibility that animals may in fact react differently to the same drugs. For instance, in examining the effects of the monoamine oxidase inhibitor SKF-385, Goldberg and Shideman (1962) found that administration of this compound lowered the concentration of catecholamines in the cat heart by about 50 to 70%, whereas the same dose increased the concentration of catecholamines in the rat heart by about 27 to 90% (see Fig. 4.1). Such inconsistencies preclude any easily formulated generalities regarding the effects of drugs. As Koppanyi and Avery (1966) point out, if penicillin had been screened in the guinea pig or Syrian hamster, both of which are affected minimally by it, this most valuable of man's chemical weapons might very well have been totally ignored.

Another rather interesting study involving the role of genetic factors concerns the consumption of alcohol by rats in a free choice situation. Voluntary alcohol consumption often has been observed to vary between different strains of rats (e.g., Reed, 1951; McClearn and Rogers, 1959); similar findings in mice have demonstrated quite convincingly that some species of rodents show definite preferences for alcohol, whereas others behave as if they were absolute "teetotalers" (McClearn and Rogers, 1959). Among the factors which have been implicated in the preference for alcohol are differences in "emotionality" and/or susceptibility to the intoxicating effects of alcohol (cf. Meier, 1963), and the "craving" or reinforcement value of alcohol (Williams, 1956).

Preliminary experiments aimed at uncovering certain physiological and/ or behavioral factors that are correlated with alcohol-drinking behavior have already been reported. One such experiment (Eriksson, 1972) involved an examination of the "open-field" behavior of two rat strains that had been bred selectively for differential alcohol consumption. The assumption behind open-field testing, which involves placing an animal in a novel environment, is that high ambulation and/ or low defecation scores are indices of an absence of fear, whereas low ambulation and high defecation

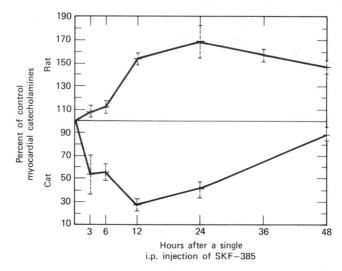

Fig. 4.1 Effects of the MAO inhibitor SKF-285 on catecholamine content of the rat and cat heart. The drug produced a marked depletion of catecholamines in the cat heart of about 70% following a dose of 12 mg/kg, an effect rather atypical of MAO inhibitors. In the rat, the usual increase in catecholamines was obtained, however (from Goldberg and Shideman, 1962).

scores are reflections of fear in animals such as the rat. The results of this study are presented in Table 4.2 The data demonstrate the feasibility of genetic selection for alcohol-drinking behavior but indicate that although there are marked differences in the consumption of alcohol between such strains, there is very little difference between them in their open-field behavior. Additional experiments along these lines, however, may uncover factors that are correlated with this genetically inherited trait (Eriksson, 1972).

Table 4.2 Relationship Between Alcohol Consumption and Open-Field Behavior[a]

Strain	Sex	Mean Daily Intake of Alcohol (g/kg)	Mean Ambulation	Mean Defecation
ANA	M	0.39	9.54	2.8
ANA	F	0.47	12.05	2.8
AA	M	7.58	7.54	2.4
AA	F	9.87	9.42	3.1

[a] Modified from Eriksson (1972).

SEX DIFFERENCES

In ascertaining the effects of drugs on the behavior of animals, one of the more obvious variables to be considered is the sex of the experimental subjects. This has been shown to be an especially important factor in toxicological studies. For example, whereas anesthetic doses of chloroform produce severe renal damage in male mice, hardly any renal deterioration occurs in females that are exposed to equivalent doses of chloroform. This difference in toxicity is related directly to the male sex hormones, since castration abolishes this difference and readministration of male hormone to castrated mice restores it (Hewitt, 1957; cf. Kato et al., 1962).

Although there are many exceptions, in general adult male animals tend to metabolize drugs at a faster rate than females (see review by Knox et al., 1956, p. 198). (See Fig. 4.2.) The enhanced activity of the hepatic enzymes in the male results from some synergistic effect of the male hormone testosterone (see Table 4.3). Whether this results in a greater sensitivity of the male to a particular drug depends upon whether the metabolites of that drug are more potent than the present compound itself.

An interesting aspect of this differential sensitivity to drugs is seen in the development of tolerance to certain drugs. For instance, although male rats develop tolerance to pentobarbital, female rats that are subjected to the identical cronic treatment exhibit no indication of having developed tolerance to this drug (Aston, 1966). Since tolerance to pentobarbital occurs as a result of the induction of enzymes responsible for its biotransforma-

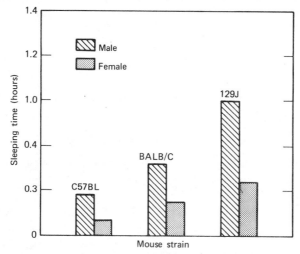

Fig. 4.2 Comparison of sleeping times induced by hexobarbital (100 mg/kg, i.p.) in three different strains of mouse (modified from Yaffe et al., 1969).

Table 4.3   Effects of Sex Hormonal Treatments on Hexobarbital Sleeping Time in Male and Female Rats[a]

Sex	Mean Sleeping Time (minutes)		
	Control	Estradiol	Testosterone
Female	90	—	38
Male	22	84	—

[a] Modified from Quinn et al. (1958).

tion, the absence of tolerance in female rats is another reflection of the differences in the efficiency of the male and female hepatic enzyme systems.

Sex differences also contribute to the manner in which drugs act on neurotransmitter systems. For instance, male cats are approximately twice as sensitive to the pressor effects of norepinephrine as are females. This differential sensitivity can be decreased by pretreating female cats with testosterone (Bhargava et al., 1967).

Another practical consideration in evaluating the effects of drugs on females is the cyclic fluctuation in blood levels of sex-related hormones. Whereas male hormonal levels after the time of sexual maturity tend to remain at a relatively constant level, female hormonal levels oscillate as a function of their estrus cycles. Such cyclic variations may affect markedly drug responsiveness as demonstrated by Yaffe et al. (1968). These investigators observed that the duration of "sleeping time" induced by hexobarbital in female $C_{57}B1$ mice is related directly to their ovulation period, the shortest "sleeping time" occurring during estrus, the longest during diestrus. An even more dramatic example of the influence of the estrus cycle on the responsiveness of females to drugs was reported by Lloyd and Pickford (1967). These experimenters found that during diestrus and anestrus when estrogenic levels are at their lowest, oxytocin acted as a vasodilator and decreased blood pressure. During estrus, however, when estrogenic levels are at their highest, oxytocin had just the opposite effect—as a result of its producing vasoconstriction, oxytocin caused an increase in blood pressure.

One relevant factor affecting hormonal levels in this regard is age. For instance, during infancy and senility the activity of many of the drug metabolizing enzymes in males and females tends to be quite similar, whereas during sexual maturity, these enzymatic differences are quite pronounced (see Table 4.4). The relationship between sexual maturity and the activity of the bodily enzymes has been reviewed thoroughly by Knox et al. (1956), the evidence being quite conclusive that the concentrations

Table 4.4 Sex Differences in Hexobarbital Sleeping Time in Rats as a Function of Age[a]

Sex	Mean Sleeping Time (minutes)			
	At Age 3 Weeks	At Age 5 Weeks	At Age 9 Weeks	At Age 14 Weeks
Males	67	31	22	19
Females	66	66	67	66

[a] Modified from Quinn et al. (1958).

and activity of these enzymes are clearly a function of the sexual maturity and the particular sex of the organism.

AGE

Young organisms often are found to be more responsive than adults to equal dosages of various drugs. In some cases, this differential sensitivity on the part of the young is due to their immaturely developed metabolic systems which are unable to inactivate drugs (see reviews by Knox et al., 1956; Driscoll and Hsia, 1958; Kretchmer, 1959; Nyland, 1966; and Kornetsky, 1970). As a result, there are often higher levels of free active drug in the bloodstream of the neonate than in that of the adult following administration of the same amount of drug. Valid comparisons between young and adult animals in terms of drug responsiveness would thus seem to necessitate in many cases a reference based on blood levels of drug, rather than administered dosage (cf. Brodie and Reid, 1971).

Another reason for the increased responsiveness of young animals to various drugs may be a result of immaturely developed blood-brain barriers compared with adults of the same species (cf. Lajtha, 1957; Bakay, 1951; and Waelsch, 1955). The evidence for the immaturity of the blood-brain barrier in the young was reviewed in Chapter 1, the implication being that a number of drugs which have difficulty in passing into the brains of older animals may do so with relative ease in the young. For example, Spooner et al. (1966) report that within 2 minutes of an intravenous injection of radioactively labeled norepinephrine, 98% of the radioactivity associated with the compound could be detected in the brains of day-old chicks compared with only 8.5% in 30-day-old chicks. Behaviorally, this differential penetrability is shown by the fact that epinephrine produces sleeplike behavior in the chick, whereas in the adult the same dose of drug produces arousal (Key and Marley, 1962).

Young animals also have been found to be affected to a much greater extent than adults by the catecholamine depleting effects of reserpine and tetrabenzine (Kulkarni and Shideman, 1966). Whereas brain catecholamine levels in infant rats remain depressed for more than 10 days after the same drug treatment (Kulkarni and Shideman, 1966).

In some instances, the greater sensitivity of the young cannot be attributed to either blood-brain barrier systems or differential activity of drug metabolizing enzymes. For example, Bianchine and Ferguson (1967) determined that the LD_{50} of sodium pentobarbital was about 30% lower in the newborn rat than that in the adult. These investigators also compared the amount of drug in the brain tissue of the animals in their experiment to see if there was any correlation between the LD_{50} and brain tissue concentration of drug. The data are presented in Table 4.5.

Table 4.5   Lethality and Toxic Brain Concentrations of Pentobarbital in Rats as a Function of Age[a]

Age (days)	Mean LD_{50} (mg/kg)	Mean Toxic Levels (μg/g) brain
<1	23	27.1
5	38	46.7
10	55	71.4
20	80	88.0
30	87	95.4
Adult	80	108.5

[a] Modified from Bianchine and Ferguson (1967).

Bianchine and Ferguson argued that if the immature blood-brain barrier of the neonatal rat plays a significant role in the greater sensitivity of the young, there ought to be a relatively higher concentration of pentobarbital in their brains compared to adult animals. The data, however, indicated that the correlation between the LD_{50} and brain tissue concentration is high for all the age groups. Consequently, it could not be argued that increased penetration of drug into the brains of the younger animals is responsible for their greater sensitivity to pentobarbital. The same reasoning would apply also to an explanation in terms of greater drug metabolizing activity in the adult. The only other alternative is that the CNS of the younger animals is basically more sensitive to this particular drug.

In addition to a greater sensitivity of the immature nervous system to certain drugs, there is evidence that it may respond differently as well. For example, chlorpromazine produces an increase in the body temperatures of young mice, but in older mice of the same sex and strain, it induces a decrease in body temperature (Bagdon and Mann, 1962).

BIOLOGICAL RHYTHMS

Gross behavior as well as physiological functioning have been observed to display rhythmic variations. For instance, it is well known that the locomotor activity of animals such as the rat and the mouse is greater at night than during the day. This increase in nocturnal muscular activity results in increased oxygen consumption and heat production and generally coincides with periods of food intake. Although changes such as these have been shown to be affected by external environmental conditions such as light and temperature, these conditions merely act to synchronize what are actually endogenous biological rhythms (Aschoff, 1965). Moreover, certain physiological mechanisms also show rhythmicity that is independent of physical activity. For example, Heusner (1956) measured the metabolic rate of rats during the night and during the day at a point when there were no differences in locomotor activity and found that there was a 25% higher metabolic rate during the daylight hours than at night, even though all measurements were conducted in darkness.

Biological rhythmicity has also been shown to constitute an important source of variability in experiments involving drug action. For example, in studying the lethality of sodium pentobarbital in mice as a function of the time of day at which the drug was administered, Lindsay and Kullman (1966) observed that lethality was greatest when the drug was injected early in the morning (7 a.m.) and least when injected at noon. In a similar kind of study, Lutsch and Morris (1967) found that lidocaine hydrochloride was about 14 times less toxic in mice if administered in the afternoon (3 p.m.) than at night (9 p.m.). Since the magnitude of the biological response to drugs is in many cases dependent upon the rate at which they are metabolized, these differences in lethality may correspond to circadian rhythms (about 24 hours) in liver enzyme activity, such as have been reported by Rapoport et al. (1966), Radzialowski and Bousquet (1968), and Wurtman and Axelrod (1967). In this regard, it should be noted also that barbiturate sleeping time, which is affected by liver enzyme activity, has been shown to be a function also of the time of day at which the drug is administered (Davis, 1962).

Circadian rhythms in the local tissue concentrations of various biogenic amines have also been reported. For example, Reis et al. (1969) have demonstrated such rhythmicity in various areas of the cat brain for norepinephrine and serotonin. Representative data from the anterior hypothalamus are presented in Fig. 4.3.

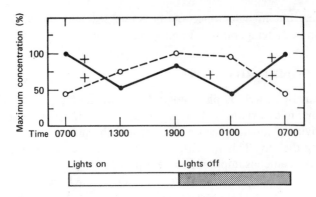

Fig. 4.3 Twenty-four-hour cycles of serotonin (●, 5-HT) and norepinephrine (○, NE) expressed as percentage of maximum 5-HT concentration in anterior hypothalamus of light-cycled cats having rhythm in both amines (from Reis et al., 1969).

Reports of a marked circadian rhythm in the serotonin content of the rat pineal gland also have appeared (e.g., Snyder et al., 1965), indicating that the pineal is not just a vestigial part of the brain as was once thought. The rhythm in the pineal gland is endogenous and still occurs in rats that have been blinded or maintained in continuous darkness (Snyder et al., 1965), but it can be influenced by laboratory lighting schedules (Snyder et al., 1967). This influence need not occur through the visual pathways, however, since external lighting conditions affect the circadian rhythm of the rat pineal gland even in infants whose eyes have not yet opened (Zweig et al., 1965).

Another aspect of biological rhythms which should not be overlooked is the seasonal variability in responsiveness to drugs (circannual rhythms). For example, a drug may produce much less of an effect during one season than another (see Fig. 4.4) because of changes in seasonal metabolic activity (cf. Nayler, 1968) or endocrine function (cf. Haus and Halberg, 1970).

The topic of biological rhythms in general is, in fact, one that is receiving more and more consideration, and there are already a fair number of books and reviews dealing with this subject (e.g., Aschoff, 1970; Halberg, 1969; Bünning, 1964; and Richter, 1965). The relationship between drugs and biological rhythmicity ("chronopharmacology") has recently been reviewed by Reinberg and Halberg (1971). In summary, it seems that studies of drug activity without reference to time parameters may result in unreliable estimations of pharmacological effects, and as a consequence potentially important drug effects may be underestimated or overlooked entirely by the unwary experimenter.

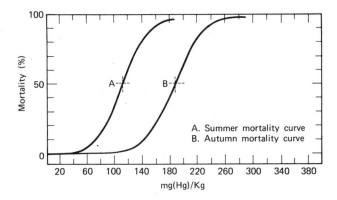

Fig. 4.4 Seasonal variation in susceptibility to toxic effects of a drug. In mice, the LD$_{50}$ of a mercurial diuretic was found to be 114 mg/kg during the summer, as compared with 187 mg/kg during the autumn (from Calesnick, 1965).

ENVIRONMENTAL TEMPERATURE

The fact that many drugs render the thermoregulatory mechanisms controlling body temperature inoperative makes the environmental temperature at the time of testing an especially critical variable in pharmacology. For instance, if an animal is no longer able to control its heat regulating mechanisms, it will become poikilothermic, and its body temperature will rise or fall according to whatever the room temperature happens to be.

Since decreases in temperature tend to slow down enzymatic reactions, a lowering of body temperature can be expected to prolong the action of any drug whose inactivation occurs by means of enzymatic degradation. For example, barbiturate drugs act to lower body temperature when animals are maintained at a room temperature below their own resting body temperature. Not surprisingly, this lowered body temperature acts to prolong the hypnotic effects of these drugs (see Table 4.6) presumably because the activity of the liver enzymes has been reduced in conjunction with this decrease in body temperature.

For most drugs that act centrally, there is a "critical ambient temperature" (Shemano and Nickerson, 1958) above which body temperature will rise and below which it will fall. By the judicious choice of an environmental temperature somewhere within this critical range, however, changes in body temperature may be prevented. Pharmacological effects due primarily to the action of the drug at its receptors can then be ascertained without a confounding of these observations by the secondary factors resulting from physiologically induced increases or decreases in body temperature.

Table 4.6   Duration of Barbiturate Sleeping Time as a Function of Room Temperature and Time of Day[a]

Temperature	Time of Day			
	10.00 a.m.	4.00 p.m.	10.00 p.m.	4.00 a.m.
26°C	90.6	122.5	82.9	66.1
36°C	58.0	57.0	60.0	41.6

[a] Modified from Davis (1962).

HOUSING CONDITIONS

One of the more subtle factors which can affect the outcome of an experiment involving drug action concerns the kind of cages animals are housed in either prior to or during an experiment. For example, if the bedding material placed in the cage to make the animal more comfortable gives off vapors that, when inhaled, stimulate enzymatic activity, then drug action may be profoundly affected. Evidence to this effect is presented in Table 4.7, which compares hexobarbital sleeping time and enzymatic activity in mice housed in cages containing either hardwood or red cedar shavings. It is apparent that sleeping time is much shorter when red cedar shavings are used as bedding material. This appears to be directly related to the effects of vapors from these shavings on the enzymes responsible for the inactivation of hexobarbital (Vesell, 1968).

Table 4.7   Duration of Hexobarbital Sleeping Time in Mice as a Function of Housing Conditions[a]

Type of Shavings	Mean Sleeping Time (minutes)
Hardwood	44
Red cedar	17

[a] Modified from Vessel (1968).

An example of the importance of housing conditions during testing comes from an experiment reported by Winter and Flataker (1962). These investigators administered morphine sulfate (s.c.) to rats and determined the mortality produced by the drug when the subjects were placed in "closed" versus "open" cages. "Closed" cages were those in which the bottom and sides were of sheet metal and the tops were of wire mesh. "Open" cages, on the other hand, were entirely of wire mesh so that there was no possibility of contact with sheet metal. The results of placing the subjects in either of these two cages are shown in Table 4.8—the mortality rate for the drug was much greater in the "closed" cage condition. Table 4.8 shows a similar effect with sodium pentobarbital as the test drug. Winter and Flataker (1962) argue that in this experiment, death occurred as a result of a combination of respiratory depression and interference with breathing produced by the sheet metal. Although the drugs produced the same extent of respiratory depression in both groups, in the closed cage condition the rat's nose became pressed against the metal sheet, and this furthered the difficulty in breathing. The investigators point out that with drugs that specifically depress respiratory function, a certain amount of attention must be paid to cage design to ensure that the animal is not deprived of air, or an entirely inaccurate estimate of drug toxicity will be obtained.

Table 4.8 Percent Mortality Following Injection of Morphine or Sodium Pentobarbital as a Function of Cage Conditions[a]

| Drug | Percent Mortality | |
	Open-Mesh Cage	Closed Metal Cage
Morphine (18.75 mg/kg)	0%	90%
Sodium pentobarbital (45 mg/kg)	8.3%	83.3%

[a] Modified from Winter and Flatakar (1962).

Indirectly related to the effect of housing conditions on drug action is the appropriateness of the test apparatus used to measure an organism's behavior. For instance, in comparing several of the different apparatuses used to measure activity in the rat, Tapp et al. (1968) were led by detailed observations of rat behavior to question seriously the validity of the assumption that all the automated apparatuses used for this purpose actually reflect spontaneous activity. The apparatuses which these investigators examined were the Williamson ("jiggle") cage, which records every movement made by the animal; the photocell cage, which records every gross movement across a photocell beam; the activity wheel, which records the number of revolutions of a wheel into which the subject is placed; a modified "open field" containing treadles which are sensitive to gross movement across them; and light contingent bar pressing, in which the animal is placed in an apparatus containing two levers, one of which produces a short light onset following its depression.

Tapp et al. (1968) argued that if activity were a unitary dimension of behavior, the intercorrelations between all measures taken from these apparatuses should be high, whereas if each apparatus were differentially sensitive to the various behaviors making up activity, the intercorrelations should be low. Their data showed that the activity scores obtained from the various apparatuses were not highly correlated, indicating that the behavior of a rat in one test situation involving activity is not at all comparable to its behavior in another, although in both cases the results are interpreted in terms of the effects of a particular manipulation on "activity." Therefore, it should not be surprising that drugs may have altogether opposite effects on "activity" when such effects are examined in different "activity" measuring devices. For example, whereas Dews (1953) reported that low doses of strychnine increase mouse activity as measured by photocell cages, both Knoll (1961) and Bastian (1961), using a tilting cage and a "motimeter" cage, respectively, reported that comparable doses of strychnine lower mouse activity. From these results, nothing can be concluded regarding the effects of strychnine on mouse activity. On the other hand, a valuable insight is apparent with respect to the problem of assessing the effects of drugs on behavior.

ENVIRONMENTAL STIMULI

The relationship between a subject's behavior and his intrinsic level of arousal or excitement has been examined by several investigators, some of whom have formulated general theories of behavior on the basis of their observations. One of the first theories of this sort was introduced by Lindsley (1950), who argued that behavior could be viewed in terms of a continuum of arousal, ranging from sleep at one end to emotional excitement at the other. This continuum, he maintained, reflects the intrinsic activity of the brain stem reticular formation. Hebb (1953) has equated the concept of "drive" with the level of arousal in the CNS and has pointed out that environmental changes such as noise, temperature, light, and the presence of others can be expected to increase the level of arousal since the neural pathways which carry information regarding these stimuli to the cortex pass through the reticular activating system.

The concept of arousal level can be extended to the effects of drugs on behavior as well, since many drugs are known to increase or decrease activity in the reticular system (see Chapter 5). Conversely, environmental changes such as those noted by Hebb ought to potentiate or attenuate drug action, depending on whether a drug increases or decreases CNS activity.

For example, it is well known that aggregation enhances the toxicity of amphetamine in mice (see Fig. 4.5). Although the mechanism by which aggregation has this effect is unknown. It is quite possible that aggregation increases amphetamine toxicity as a result of the increase in CNS excitation that arises from the mutual stimulation of each of the animals in the group. The fact that increases in noise level and temperature also act to increase the toxicity of amphetamine in isolated mice (Chance, 1947) suggests than any environmental factors which increase the level of arousal in the CNS can be expected ot modify the effects of drugs on behavior.

SPECIES-SPECIFIC BEHAVIOR

As recently pointed out by Bolles (1969), some kinds of behavior are acquired more readily (cf. Walters and Abel, 1970) and/or are more resistant to extinction than others because they have greater significance for the survival of the species. Consideration of the kinds of behavior being demanded of an organism can also have important bearing on the behavioral assessment of drugs. For example, chlorpromazine and chlordiazepoxide have been observed to increase the aggressive behavior of a

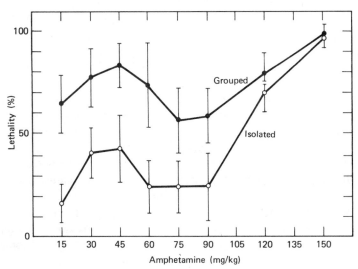

Fig. 4.5 Mean Toxicity of amphetamine (i.p.) in grouped versus isolated mice (modified from Mennear and Rudzik, 1965).

carnivorous and predatory strain of mouse (*Onychomys leucogaster*) but decrease the same kind of behavior in a nonpredatory strain (Cole and Wolf, 1966). In a similar vein, chlorpromazine has been observed to have much less of a suppressant effect on avoidance behavior which involves the performance of a genetically predisposed arboreal response than it has on a relatively arbitrarily imposed terrestrial response for the woodland deer mouse, *Peromyscus maniculatus gracilis* (Wolf et al., 1962).

The effects of several central depressant drugs on arboreal and terrestrial avoidance behavior in the prairie deer mouse, *p. m. bairdi,* have also been studied (Cole and Wolf, 1969). For the "arboreal" response, the subjects were required to remain on a threaded Plexiglas pole which had been placed at grid level at the far end of an electrified shuttle box. For the "terrestrial" response, the Plexiglas pole was replaced with a wooden pan. A conditioned response was said to have occurred when the subject mounted the pole or pan within 5 seconds of the onset of a buzzer (conditioned stimulus). The results indicated that each of the drugs tested (chlorpromazine, chlordiazepoxide, meprobamate, and sodium pentobarbital) had much less of an effect when avoidance involved a "terrestrial" response than in the case of avoidance involving an "arboreal" response. Since *p. m. bairdi* is a terrestrial mouse strain for which an arboreal response is quite foreign to its normal behavioral repetoire, this experiment demonstrates that responses that are part of a subject's natural activity tend to be much more resistant to the effects of drugs than are responses that are imposed arbitrarily upon an organism.

PRIOR EXPERIENCE

The familiarity of the subject with the test situation has on numerous occasions been found to modify drug action. For example, in one experiment Bainbridge (1970) placed mice in an activity cage immediately after injecting them with amphetamine and compared their behavior with another group of mice given the same amount of drug but exposed to the activity cage for an hour before being injected. Control animals for each of these treatments received saline injections. All animals were then tested for 1 hour. The results indicated that amphetamine acted to reduce the activity of those mice that had been tested immediately after being injected but had had no prior exposure to the apparatus, whereas it acted to increase the activity of those animals that had been exposed previously to the test situation. Similar results have also been reported for rats under somewhat different test conditions (Rushton and Steinberg, 1963).

Familiarity with the test situation has also been shown to affect the development of tolerance to the analgesic effects of morphine in rats tested with the hot plate procedure. In one such study by Gebhart et al. (1971), male Holtzman rats received either saline or morphine sulfate (10 mg/kg) and were tested on the hot plate immediately before drug administration and 30 minutes after receiving the drug. A response was defined as either a licking of the paws or jumping up the side of the test cylinder. Analgesia was defined in terms of an increased latency for either of these responses. Animals were treated in this manner for four consecutive days. A second group received identical drug treatment but no exposure to the test apparatus. On the fifth day all subjects were drugged and tested on the hot plate. In addition, a number of animals that had been injected previously with saline but had had no prior exposure to the apparatus were also injected with morphine and tested. The analgesic effects of morphine were found to be much lower in both groups of chronically treated subjects, indicating that tolerance to the drug had occurred in both conditions. However, for those chronically treated morphine subjects that were exposed to the hot plate for the first time, the reaction time was significantly higher (= greater analgesia) than it was for those subjects that had been exposed repeatedly to the apparatus prior to testing. Thus brief exposures to the test situation can significantly affect the actions of drugs in several ways, an important factor to keep in mind if animals are to be tested repeatedly (cf. Rushton and Steinberg, 1963).

In some instances, the influence of past experience may take the form of the husbandry conditions to which animals have been subjected (cf. Denenberg and Wimbey, 1963). The literature dealing with the effects of "handling" unquestionably illustrates how seemingly innocuous treatments such as picking up a subject prior to testing may have important ramifications for its subsequent behavior (see review by Thompson and Grusec, 1970), although the explanation for this effect is still a matter of uncertainty (cf. Abel, 1970).

The circumstances under which a response is learned has also been shown by Terrace (1963) to be a rather important variable affecting the action of drugs on behavior. For instance, in a typical discrimination problem, the subject has to learn the direct his responses to one of two or more stimuli. The usual procedure is to present both stimuli to the subject and to reward only the "appropriate" choice. In such situations, the subject responds on a random basis making many errors until he learns which stimulus-response contingencies lead to reinforcement and which go unrewarded. However, during this kind of learning the subject often relapses and responds to the incorrect stimulus, and this occasionally precipitates some kind of "emotional" response. Using a "fading" procedure, involving the presentation of a brightly illuminated positive stimulus (S_+) along with a dimly lighted negative stimulus (S_-) and rewarding the pigeon's greater tendency to peck the more brightly illuminated of the two, Terrace has shown that as training progresses, he can increase the brightness of the negative stimulus ("fading in") until eventually both stimuli are of equal brightness. Under such conditions, the pigeon continues to peck only the reinforced stimulus and thus the discrimination has been learned with virtually no errors.

After training a number of pigeons under one of these two kinds of discrimination procedures, that is, with and without errors, Terrace (1963) has administered either chlorpromazine, imipramine, or saline to his subjects every third day and observed the effects of these drugs on performance. As shown in Table 4.9, neither chlorpromazine nor imipramine has any effect on the performance of the pigeons that have learned the discrimination without errors. Conversely, both drugs dramatically increase the number of responses to the negative stimulus for those animals that have learned the discrimination with errors. Neither drug, however, has any effect on the frequency of responding to the positive stimulus (S_+). Terrace's (1963) work thus constitutes another example of the way in which the prior experience of a subject can influence markedly the actions of a drug on its behavior.

Prior learning has been shown to affect drug action in other ways as well. For instance, animals that have already learned to make an avoidance

Table 4.9 Effects of Chlorpromazine and Imipramine on Key-Pecking Performance as a Function of Training Conditions[a]

	Mean Responses to S_-	
Dose (mg/kg)	Trained "Without Errors"	Trained "With Errors"
Chlorpromazine		
1	0	92.5
3	0	607
10	0	802
17	0	2678
Imipramine		
1	0	415.5
3	0	867.5
10	0	2580.5
17	0	5471

[a] Modified from Terrace (1963).

response are much more resistant to drugs that suppress avoidance behavior than are those that have not completely learned such avoidance behavior (Irwin, 1960). Similarly, rats that have thoroughly learned a barpressing response are affected by drugs to a much less extent than are less experienced subjects. In general, drugs tend to have less of an effect on already learned material than on to-be-learned material in humans as well (cf. Abel, 1971).

Habit strength and motivational level are additional variables that must be considered. For example, Singh and Manocha (1966) have demonstrated that both overlearning and increased "drive" level will attenuate the suppressive effects of drugs on behavior. In an illustrative experiment, rats were trained in a lever-pressing situation (water reward) until the subjects attained a predetermined criterion of responses per session. The animals were then divided into three groups, two of which were given additional periods of overtraining. The animals in each of these groups were subdivided further shortly before the test session into three "drive" level groups according to the number of hours of water deprivation to which they had tested after receiving either chlorpromazine or a placebo. The experiment revealed that when behavior is well established and performed under high levels of motivation, it is much more resistant to the effects of drugs than when it is poorly established and performed under conditions of low motivation.

PREDRUG LEVELS OF ONGOING ACTIVITY

An important determinant of the behavioral effects of a drug is the frequency of occurrence of the behavior being recorded. This relationship between predrug rates of responding and drug action has been referred to as the "law of initial value" (Wilder, 1957) or "rate dependency" (cf. Kelleher and Morse, 1969). Briefly stated, these concepts propose that the higher the "initial level" of rate of responding, the smaller the effect of excitatory drugs, and the greater the effect of depressant drugs on that behavior. Conversely, the lower the initial level or response rate, the greater the effect of excitatory and the smaller the effect of depressant drugs.

Wilder (1957) has argued that the relationship between drug effects and control rates of responding follows the Weber-Fechner law of psychophysics relating sensation and perception. According to Wilder, as "initial values" increase arithmetically, response rates to drugs increase geometrically, and he has amassed a sizable body of physiological data in support of his proposal. More recently, an impressive number of studies have appeared which show that with some drugs, "initial values" likewise influence the direction of behavioral change.

One of the earliest of such studies was reported by Dews (1958), who administered methamphetamine to pigeons working for food under different schedules of reinforcement, two of which induced a relatively high rate of responding whereas the other two generated a relatively low response rate. Dews found that the same low doses of methamphetamine increased the rate of responding on the schedules generating the low response rates but decreased behavior on those generating high response rates.

MOTIVATIONAL LEVEL

Rather than examining the control rate of responding as a variable affecting the behavioral response to various drugs, Hill et al. (1957) have focused on the incentives that serve to generate either high or low rates of responding and have investigated how these incentives act to modify drug action. Employing a simple visual-manual reaction-time situation, Hill et al. found that morphine addicts who were offered a small incentive for performing the experimental task manifested a typical depression in behavior when treated with pentobarbital. However, if the incentive was high (e.g., an injection of morphine), pentobarbital acted to shorten significantly their reaction times. In other words, pentobarbital had a facilitating effect on their performance under the high incentive condition. Thus, depending upon the incentives motivating behavior, drugs such as pentobarbital may increase, decrease, or have no effect at all upon behavior (see Table 4.10).

This alternative to the "rate-dependency" explanation may help to explain a rather interesting exception to the rate-dependency effect of amphetamine, namely, that low rates of responding that are maintained by electric shock are not increased by amphetamine (Kelleher and Morse, 1968). With respect to morphine, an effect similar to that of amphetamine has been reported by Edwards (1961), who showed that whereas it re-

Table 4.10 Effects of Motivational Level on Performance Following Injection of Morphine or Pentobarbital[a]

	Reaction Time	
Drug Condition	Low Incentive	High Incentive
Control	206	171
Morphine	188	171
Pentobarbital	233	160

[a] Modified from Hill et al. (1957).

quired 0.37 mg/kg of morphine to suppress behavior that was appetitively motivated (food reward), it required more than 10 times that amount (5.9 mg/kg) of morphine to suppress behavior that was motivated by an aversive stimulus. The incentives that are attached to the performance of a particular task thus constitute another important variable to consider in evaluating the interaction between drugs and behavior.

5. Pharmacology of the CNS

THE PROBLEM OF CLASSIFICATION

The growth of any science is characterized by the description of pertinent phenomena followed by the grouping and classifying of these descriptions into meaningful categories. Only by placing the hundreds and thousands of individual pieces of relevant information into some meaningful schemata can scientists ever hope to make abstractions and generalizations concerning the laws governing their fields of interest. This is, of course, one of the important *sine qua nons* for continued growth and development. This fact is clearly evident in comparing the lasting contributions of the ancient civilizations of the world. The civilization of ancient Egypt, for example, preceded that of the Greeks by several centuries. During this interim the Egyptians accumulated many facts and, in many cases, developed these facts into practical applications. But it was the Greeks who first saw the necessity for classifying information so that generalizations and laws of nature could be formulated (Abel, 1973); as a result, it is to the Greeks that we owe our own scientific heritage and accomplishments.

In classifying information, one of the first problems that must be solved is agreeing on the criteria for classification. As an indication of the inherent difficulties involved in such a basic problem, Ray (1972) has outlined some of the different categories to which the drug amphetamine might be assigned by various professionals if the classification fell to them. By the physician, for example, amphetamine might be identified as an antiappetite drug because it decreases the food intake of his patients for a time. The lawyer, on the other hand, would probably look upon it as a drug of abuse which falls under Schedule II of the 1970 Federal drug laws. By the psychologist, it might be regarded as a stimulant; by the chemist, as a phenylethylamine; and the user himself would probably identify it as an "upper." To the pharmacologist, the problem is even more acute because in pharmacology, a primary objective is the identification of the mechanism of action of drugs and as yet, this is still largely unknown in the case of amphetamine and many of the other drugs with which he works. This difficulty is especially compounded by the fact that many drugs act indirectly, so that no simple classification such as those of his colleagues in other disciplines will apply to his own.

For example, if a drug causes behavioral excitation, this effect may be caused by direct stimulation of excitatory neural centers, a lowering of the threshold to excitatory stimuli, a raising of the threshold for inhibitory impulses, or a suppression of the neural activity in inhibitory centers. Conversely, behavior may be depressed as a result of the direct stimulation of inhibitory centers, direct inhibition of excitatory centers, an increase in the threshold for the stimulation of excitatory neurons, or a decrease in the threshold of neurons that carry inhibitory impulses.

The main difficulty is thus one of specifying the primary site of drug action and one of the main reasons for the unsatisfactory classification of drugs at present is our ignorance of the location of these sites (as well as their mechanisms of action at either the cellular or the molecular level). Were such information available, pharmacologists would possess a sound practical, if not theoretical, basis on which to erect a meaningful schemata for classifying drugs and their effects (Toman, 1962).

To illustrate this problem further, consider the effects of the drug strychnine. At low doses strychnine increases motor activity whereas at high doses it induces convulsions. In light of these behavioral effects, strychnine is often characterized as a stimulant. However, the mechanism of action of this drug involves a blocking of the activity of specific inhibitory neurons that are located in the spinal column (Eccles et al., 1963; Fuortes and Nelson, 1963). How then should strychnine be classified—as a stimulant because of its behavioral effects, or a depressant because of its mechanism of action?

The problem that immediately arises with placing compounds that produce similar behavioral effects in the same category regardless of their mechanisms of action is thus one of determining whether there are any behavioral effects produced by drugs that are specific enough to distinguish one compound from another. If this can be done, then the next step is to try to determine whether these behavioral effects have any unique neurophysiological and/or neurochemical correlates. The solution to these problems has taken a number of different directions, but at present the most promising seems to be that of using the techniques of the psychologist to identify both the specific behavioral effects of drugs and the physiological basis of their activity.

For example, one approach used by the psychologist to identify the neuroanatomical correlates of behavior involves examining the effects on behavior resulting from electrical stimulation of circumscribed areas of the brain. In the case of food intake, for example, this procedure has demonstrated reliably that stimulation of the lateral areas of the hypothalamus causes a satiated animal to eat voraciously. On the other hand, electrical stimulation of the ventromedial area of the hypothalamus has been shown to inhibit eating in a very hungry animal. Once these neuroanatomical sites were identified, recording electrodes were implanted in these same areas and the neurophysiological correlates of hunger and satiety were determined. The observations arising out of these techniques have now led to the identification of these two areas as the probable centers for hunger and satiety, respectively, in the brain. This phenomenon also has been studied by injecting chemicals directly into the brain by means of implanted cannulae. Since the results of these studies are discussed at great length shortly, no more is said about them here except to note that an approach such as this offers a means of identifying the neurochemical correlates of behavior; by using this technique, it has become possible to identify drugs in terms of whether they mimic or antagonize the actions of some suspected neurotransmitter.

In addition to these neurophysiological and neurochemical behavioral procedures, there are also a number of test situations in which behavioral measures are used as dependent variables which permit the psychopharmacologist, or behavioral pharmacologist as he is otherwise known, to identify drugs that may have potentially useful clinical applications. One such test procedure that appears to do just that is the conditioned avoidance technique.

Conditioned avoidance is a situation in which a signal is presented to an animal which warns it of the imminence of an aversive stimulus such as electric shock. After a number of signal-shock pairings, the animal typically learns to make some response such as running from one compartment of the test apparatus to another when the signal is presented, in order to avoid the shock. If the animal responds to the signal prior to the delivery of shock, he is said to have made a conditioned active avoidance response. On the other hand, if he moves from the shock compartment to the non-shock area only in reaction to the shock, he is said to have made an unconditioned escape response. Studying the effect of drugs on this procedure involves determining whether a particular agent differentially affects the conditioned avoidance response without affecting escape behavior. A general property of the antipsychotic (major tranquilizer) drugs is that they do in fact reduce conditioned avoidance behavior at doses that do not affect unconditioned responding. By comparison, sedative-hypnotic drugs such as the barbiturates suppress both conditioned and unconditioned behavior in such test situations. Because of the reliability of this technique in identifying potentially useful antipsychotic drugs, it has become a standard screening test in psychopharmacology. However, the relationship between suppression of conditioned avoidance behavior and psychotic behavior is difficult to discern and for this reason this test has been criticized on the grounds that it lacks face validity.

In keeping with these two general approaches to the study of drug action, namely, elucidating the neurochemical correlates of behavior and identifying drugs with chemically useful applications, the first part of the following discussion deals with those compounds whose behavioral effects can be accounted for on the basis of whether they mimic or inhibit the activity of transmitter mechanisms in the CNS. This is then followed by several illustrations of how these drugs have been employed as tools in the pharmacological analysis of behavior. Following this, the discussion turns to a consideration of drugs commonly employed in clinical situations and to some of their possible mechanisms of action.

PHARMACOLOGY OF THE CHOLINERGIC SYNAPSE

Acetylcholine (ACh) has long been recognized as the neurochemical mediating synaptic transmission in the peripheral nervous system at preganglionic nerve endings in both sympathetic and parasympathetic fibers, at the postganglionic endings in functionally parasympathetic fibers, and at the neuromuscular junctions at striated (voluntary) muscles. As pointed out in Chapter 1, acetylcholine is also present in the CNS and although its function in this area has not been settled unequivocally, it seems fairly certain that it acts as a neurotransmitter in the brain and the cerebrospinal system as well. Consequently, any substance able to affect the activity of the cholinergic system will undoubtedly have profound effects on behavior. This could occur readily if a drug were to influence (1) the synthesis, (2) storage, or (3) release of the transmitter substance, or if it were to (4) directly stimulate cholinergic receptors, (5) block these receptors, or (6) interfere with the inactivation of the transmitter, thus causing the duration of action of the transmitter at its receptor sites to be prolonged. The following commentary deals with some of the drugs which have been used more commonly to influence these events at the cholinergic synapse.

Interference with the Synthesis of ACh

Acetylcholine is synthesized from choline and acetate by the enzyme choline acetylase, and it is then stored for future use at the nerve endings. At present, there are only a few substances that are able to interfere with the synthesis of ACh and of these, hemicholinium (HC-3) is the most potent. This interference is brought about by the inhibition of the mechanism which transports choline into cholinergic fibers. The result of this inhibition is a reduction of ACh levels in synaptic boutons, thus preventing the transmission of impulses in cholinergically mediated fibers. However, this paralysis of function is confined mainly to the peripheral nervous system since hemicholinium does not readily penetrate the blood-brain barrier.

Interference with Storage of Transmitter

Although a number of compounds have been developed for the purpose of depleting norepinephrine from its storage sites, hardly any compounds have been synthesized for the purpose of producing the same kind of interference in cholinergic pathways.

Interference with Transmitter Release

Few compounds have been synthesized for the purpose of preventing the release of ACh from cholinergic fibers. However, a naturally occurring substance which produces this kind of effect is the *botulinus* toxin which has been implicated in many cases of food poisoning. In such cases, death may occur as a result of respiratory paralysis due to the prevention of acetylcholine release from neural pathways involved in breathing.

Interference with Cholinomimetics

The central effects of ACh cannot be observed if this compound is administered by the usual systemic routes since ACh is a quaternary ammonium compound and consequently, because of the presence of the positively charged ammonium group in its structure, it does not readily penetrate the blood-brain barrier. Moreover, ACh is destroyed rapidly by the cholinesterases found in the bloodstream. However, by altering the ACh molecule, new compounds have been produced which resemble ACh in their activity and which have the added characteristic of being more resistant to the effects of the cholinesterases. This enables them to enter the brain more readily following systemic administration and extends their duration of activity in the central nervous system. These drugs, whose chief characteristic is that they imitate the interaction between endogenously released ACh and its postsynaptic receptors, are termed cholinomimetics.

One such compound in this series is methacholine. This drug is completely resistant to degradation by butyrocholinesterase and is much more resistant to inactivation by acetylcholinesterase than is acetylcholine. Carbachol (carbamylcholine), however, is the most potent of all the cholinomimetics, being quite resistant to inactivation by both types of cholinesterases. The activity of methacholine and carbachol relative to ACh as measured by their effects on rabbit blood pressure is presented in Table 5.1. Additional compounds of this type are urecholine and furtrethonium. However, these cholinomimetics are not encountered often in behavioral research.

Table 5.1 Comparison of Pharmacological Potency of Methacholine and Carbachol Relative to Acetylcholine[a]

Compound	Relative Activity (ACh = 1)		
	i.v.	s.c.	Oral
Acetylcholine	1	1	1
Methacholine	1	5	20
Carbachol	1	10	500

[a] Modified from Molitor (1936).

Before leaving the cholinomimetics, mention also should be made of three naturally occurring substances which in various ways mimic the action of ACh. These are nicotine, muscarine, and pilocarpine. The former two are found in tobacco and certain mushrooms (*Amanita muscaria*), respectively. In mice, the lethality of muscarine is approximately 100 times greater than that of acetylcholine (Volle, 1971) and it is well known that muscarine-containing mushrooms may cause death if they are eaten inadvertently. The third naturally occurring cholinomimetic is pilocarpine, which is found in the leaves of the plant *Pilocarpus juborandi*.

Interference with the Inactivation of ACh

A number of compounds are able to potentiate the effects of ACh by their inhibition of the activity of the cholinesterases. These anticholinesterases (anti-ChEs) may also be administered to potentiate the effects of cholinomimetic compounds such as methacholine and carbachol. Since anticholinesterases act to raise the levels of ACh at cholinergic synapses by preventing the destruction of the transmitter, they too may produce behavioral effects resembling those of ACh, and hence they are conceptually similar to the cholinomimetic agents.

Two of the more commonly employed anticholinesterases used in behavioral research are physostigmine (eserine) and neostigmine. The mechanism of action of these compounds involves their competition with ACh for the surface of the enzyme, acetylcholinesterase, at which ACh is normally inactivated. Physostigmine, which readily penetrates the blood-brain barrier, may be administered by the general systemic routes if its actions on central cholinergic mechanisms are of interest. However, systemic administration will deliver this drug to peripheral sites as well, and it may not be possible to distinguish the central from the peripheral effects of this drug. One possibility for distinguishing between the central and peripheral effects of the anti-ChEs is to compare the effects of physostigmine with those of neostigmine. The latter contains a quaternary ammonium nitrogen in its structure and therefore it does not readily penetrate the blood-brain barrier. Hence its actions are confined chiefly to the peripheral nervous system.

Physostigmine and neostigmine are also termed reversible cholinesterase inhibitors because they form a transient complex with this enzyme and hence their effects last for only a few hours. There are a number of other anticholinesterases, however, whose duration of action is much longer. Two of these substances presently used in many agricultural pesticides are diisopropylfluorophosphate (DFP) and parathion. These anticholinesterases are termed irreversible because their actions cannot be altered directly.

Blockade of the Effects of ACh

Although cholinergic receptors are all sensitive to ACh, the pharmacological characteristics of all the ACh-sensitive receptors are not the same. For instance, drugs that mimic the effects of ACh at one cholinergic receptor may have markedly attenuated effects at another. Similarly, drugs that block cholinergic transmission at one cholinergic receptor may have no blocking action at another. It is as a result of such observations that Dale (1914) distinguished between the muscarinelike and nicotinelike actions of ACh. As a consequence of this distinction, cholinergic blocking compounds, termed anticholinergics or cholinolytics, are dichotomized into those which act at muscarinic and those which act as nicotinic receptors.

MUSCARINIC ANTICHOLINERGICS

Antimuscarinic compounds are sometimes termed atropinic since atropine is the prototype of this series. Closely related to atropine in activity, however, is scopolamine. Both are naturally occurring alkaloids of the belladonna plant ("deadly nightshade"). The anticholinergic activity of these substances does not involve their preventing the release of ACh from nerve endings but rather appears to involve their occupation of certain cholinergic receptors in such a way that they prevent the naturally occurring transmitter from gaining access to these receptors. However, neither atropine nor scopolamine initiates any response following combination with these ACh-sensitive receptors. Their predominant effect is instead that of preventing ACh from producing any response. Neither atropine nor scopolamine, however, has any blocking action at nicotinic sites. In fact, so selective are the actions of these compounds in blocking the effects of ACh at muscarinic receptors that they are often administered in conjunction with other drugs to determine whether the latter have any muscarinic activity. Thus if atropine is able to block the agonist effects of a particular drug, it is assumed that the site of action of that agonist is a muscarine-like receptor.

Both atropine and scopolamine readily penetrate the blood-brain barrier. However, when administered systematically, they can also produce peripheral effects which may be difficult to differentiate from their central actions. To distinguish between these two sites of action, the effects of these compounds are sometimes contrasted with those of methylatropine and methscopolamine, respectively. The attachment of these methyl groups to the parent compounds acts to convert them into quaternary ammonium compounds which do not enter into the central nervous system. Comparing the behavioral effects of these methylated compounds with their parent substances is thus one way of identifying the primary site of action underlying the behavioral effects of these drugs.

NICOTINIC ANTICHOLINERGICS.

In contrast to muscarinic receptors, nicotinic receptors are subdivided into two subgroups since there are some nicotinic anticholinergics which selectively block transmission in autonomic ganglia and others which selectively block neuromuscular transmission.

The protoype of the nicotinic blocking drugs acting at autonomic sites is hexamethonium. Like atropine, this compound blocks cholinergic transmission by occupying cholinergic receptors, thus preventing the access of the transmitter to these sites. Hexamethonium has no blocking action at muscarinic or at neuromuscular receptor sites, however.

Typical of those drugs which act by combining with nicotine-sensitive receptors at neuromuscular sites is *d*-tubocurarine (curare). In doing so, this compound interferes with the ability of ACh to act at these receptors resulting in the paralysis of voluntary muscle. Gallamine (Flaxedil) is another neuromuscular blocking agent whose actions are similar to those of d-tubocurarine, but it is much less potent than the latter. Two other neuromuscular blocking compounds are decamethonium and succinyl-choline, but their mode of action is much different from that of d-tubo-curarine and gallamine. Instead of preventing ACh from combining with its receptors, they cause the depolarization of postsynaptic skeletal muscle membranes for prolonged periods of time, thus rendering neuromuscular transmission inoperative until the drug can be metabolized or removed from the neuromuscular junction by diffusion.

Following this review of the pharmacology of the cholinergic system, the evidence implicating this system in the phenomenon of thirst is presented. To facilitate discussion of this subject matter, Table 5.2 summarizes much of the material just presented.

Table 5.2   Summary of Compounds Acting at the Cholinergic Synapse

Site of Action	Compound	Effect
Interference with synthesis of ACh	Hemicholinium	Anticholinergic
Interference with release of ACh	Botulinus toxin	Anticholinergic
Stimulation of postsynaptic receptors		
Muscarinic	Carbachol, methacholine	Cholinomimetic
Nicotinic	Nicotine	Cholinomimetic
Blockade of postsynaptic receptors		
Muscarinic	Atropine, scopolamine	Anticholinergic
Nicotinic	Hexamethonium	Anticholinergic
	d-Tubocurarine	Anticholinergic
Interference with enzymatic inactivation	Physostigmine	Cholinomimetic
	Neostigmine	Cholinomimetic

CHOLINERGIC MEDIATION OF WATER INTAKE

Behavioral studies involving the application of acetylcholine to brain tissue have given rise to a rather impressive body of literature supporting the involvement of this substance as the neurochemical mediating behavior in certain neural pathways. This information is of importance both from the point of view of the mechanisms underlying various behavioral activities and from the standpoint of offering a tool for the testing of drugs for their possible cholinergic activity in the CNS. It may be recalled from the discussion in Chapter 1, however, that the behavior of cholinergic cells in the CNS in response to topical applications of ACh is quite different from the response of peripherally located cholinergic neurons when treated in the same manner. For instance, it has been shown that ACh produces depolarizations in cortical neurons without altering their membrane resistance (Krnjević and Schwartz, 1967). In addition, although most cortical neurons respond to ACh with increased rates of firing, the latency of onset for this response is quite slow and the duration of excitation is relatively long, compared with the onset and duration of ACh when it is applied to peripheral neurons (Krnjević and Phillis, 1963; Krnjević et al., 1971). The fact that the administration of acetylcholine elicits specific kinds of behavior when applied to circumscribed areas in the brain, however, indicates that despite these anomalies, acetylcholine does seem to play some part in CNS activity. The pharmacological aspects of this involvement are now presented with respect to the thirst mechanism in the brain.

It is generally agreed that the hypothalamus exerts a controlling influence over food and water intake, since animals with lesions in this part of the brain refuse to take food or water (Teitelbaum and Stellar, 1954). The fact that both food and water intake are abolished by the same small bilateral lesions suggests that the neural pathways involved in these activities are coexistent in the hypothalamus. However, on the basis of chemical stimulation studies pioneered by Grossman (1960, 1962a, 1962b) it has been shown that these anatomically coexistent pathways can be differentiated on the basis of chemical substances introduced into this area of the brain. Evidence that adrenergic chemicals are able to elicit feeding behavior when applied to the lateral hypothalamus is reviewed in a later section. In this section, the evidence linking fluid intake with stimulation of cholinergic pathways is presented.

A cholinergically mediated system underlying water intake has been proposed as a result of the observation that injections of acetylcholine into the lateral hypothalamus of the rat elicit drinking in satiated animals. When carbachol is used instead of acetylcholine, drinking behavior is also elicited, the duration of action being prolonged owing to the fact that carbachol is poorly hydrolyzed by cholinesterase. The nature and specificity of this effect is illustrated in Fig. 5.1. In general, drinking begins 2 to 3 minutes after injection of these substances and lasts for about 20 to 30 minutes, the amount of water being consumed being about 0.5 ml/min.

The effect itself appears to be specifically mediated by muscarinic receptors since it occurs in response to muscarine but not to nicotine (Stein and Seifter, 1962). The specificity of this cholinergic mediation of drink-

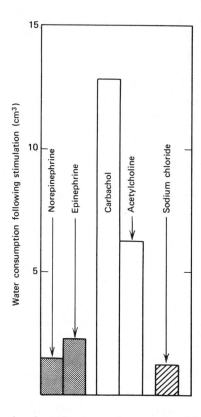

Fig. 5.1 Water intake during the first hour following chemical stimulation of the lateral hypothalamus of the rat. Administration of acetylcholine and carbachol in this area resulted in dramatic increases in water consumption. Injection of adrenergic substances resulted in significantly less drinking, demonstrating that the effect was not due to non-specific activation. Similarly, administration of sodium chloride to this area was also without effect, showing that osmotic stimulation was not a factor in the elicitation of drinking by these cholinergic substances (from Gorssman, 1960).

ing has also been demonstrated by the fact that (1) the amount of water consumed is dose dependent (see Fig. 5.2); (2) other biogenic amines do not elicit drinking (see Fig. 5.1); (3) systematic injections of atropine are able to inhibit the water intake typically produced by cholinomimetic agents (see Fig. 5.3); and (4) the central administration of anticholinesterase agents such as eserine act to potentiate drinking behavior in water-deprived rats.

A further indication that this effect is centrally mediated is evident from the fact that scopolamine and atropine both suppress drinking in water-deprived rats whereas the methyl quaternary analogues of these compounds (which penetrate the blood-brain barrier with difficulty) do not (see Table 5.3).

Following Grossman's original report of drinking produced by cholinergic stimulation of lateral hypothalamic nuclei, Fisher and Coury (1962) "mapped" the cholinergic pathway mediating water intake in the rat and found a very close correlation between the areas from which cholinergically induced drinking could be obtained and parts of the Papez (1937)

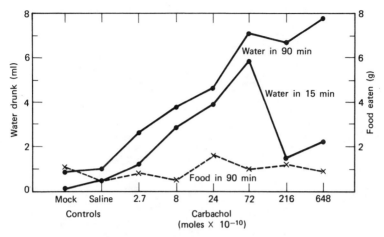

Fig. 5.2 Effects of different doses of carbachol in ventromedial nucleus of hypothalamus on eating and drinking (from Miller et al., 1964).

Table 5.3 Effects of Anticholinergic Drugs on Water Consumption in Water-Deprived (23 Hours) Rats[a]

Compound	Dose (mg/kg)	Mean Water Consumption (ml)
Saline	—	20.2
Scopolamine	0.4	10.3
Scopolamine	0.8	6.3
Scopolamine methyl nitrate	0.4	18.8
Scopolamine methyl nitrate	0.8	15.7
Atropine	2.5	17.3
Atropine	5.0	12.5
Atropine methyl nitrate	5.0	17.0

[a] Adapted from Stein (1963).

motivational circuit. Recently, it has been argued that this circuit underlies many innate activities such as sex, fight-flight, and consummatory behavior (Papez, 1959). It is thus possible that chemical stimulation of this circuit may activate pathways that pass through the lateral hypothalamus on the way to effector mechanisms involved in drinking behavior.

Evidence that cholinergic stimulation of the lateral hypothalamus does have motivational properties is suggested by the observation that rats trained to press one bar for food and another for water press the latter

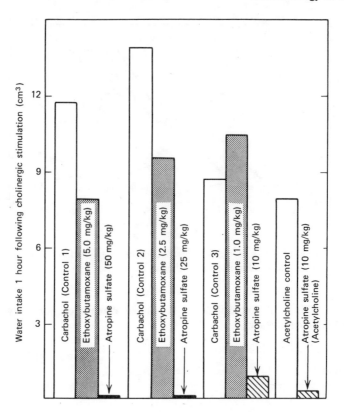

Fig. 5.3   Antagonism of carbachol-induced drinking by systemic injections of atropine. The adrenergic blocking compound ethoxybutamoxane has a slight but probably nonspecific effect. Blocking compounds were injected (i.p.) 1 hour before central administration of carbachol (from Grossman, 1962*b*).

when cholinergically stimulated (see Fig. 5.4). Likewise cholinergic stimulation of the same area has been shown to motivate the acquisition and continued performance of maze learning for water reinforcement as effectively as does $23\frac{1}{2}$ hours of water deprivation (Khavari and Russel, 1966). Observations such as these preclude the possibility that the effects of cholinergic stimulation are due solely to the activation of effector mechanisms involved in drinking behavior.

In summary, drinking has been elicited reliably by intracranial administrations of acetycholine and carbachol (a cholinomimetic compound). Eserine (a cholinesterase inhibitor) potentiates drinking following water deprivation, whereas atropine (a cholinergic blocking agent) reduces drinking somewhat following water deprivation. Investigations of the various

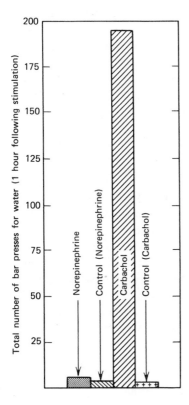

Fig. 5.4 Effects of cholinergic and adrenergic stimulation of the lateral hypothalamus of satiated rats on bar pressing for water reward. Control levels were determined during a 1-hour period preceding each stimulation. These results demonstrate that chemical stimulation of this area has motivational properties resembling the effects of water deprivation. These effects are specifically related ot cholinergic stimulation since adrenergically stimulated rats did not press a bar for water (from Grossman, 1962b).

areas of the brain that are responsive to cholinergic manipulation have suggested that the cholinergic pathway mediating thirst is homologous to the Papez limbic-hypothalamic circuit. In addition, carbachol-induced thirst possesses some of the same motivational characteristics associated with water deprivation.

However, in contrast to this rather impressive body of data linking thirst to activity in certain cholinergic pathways of the brain, the conclusion that the fluid intake induced by cholinomimetic agents is similar to that produced following water deprivation is still somewhat conjectural. For one thing, carbachol-induced drinking has been demonstrated only in rats. Comparable results have not been observed when similar techniques and areas of the brain have been investigated in cats, rabbits, or monkeys (Fisher and Coury, 1964; Myers, 1964, 1969). This suggests that the phenomenon of carbachol-induced drinking in rats may be species-specific. Secondly, although atropine does inhibit carbachol-induced drinking, it only partially inhibits drinking following water deprivation. Finally, there is also a difference between carbachol-induced drinking and drinking induced by water deprivation in terms of preference or aversion for liquids, for example, alcohol (Cicero and Myers, 1969). Thus, although pharmacological manipulations of the brain have elucidated one of the cholinergic mechanisms that may underlie thirst in the rat,.it appears that much more still remains to be discovered concerning the neurological mechanisms involved in thirst. Pharmacological manipulations, however, offer one promising approach to this problem.

PHARMACOLOGY OF THE ADRENERGIC SYNAPSE

According to the terminology of Barger and Dale (1910), drugs that elicit physiological responses similar to those observed consequent to stimulation of the sympathetic nervous system are designated "sympathomimetic." Since the chemical transmitter at this division of the autonomic nervous system is norepinephrine, the term sympathomimetic implies a resemblance to the physiological effects of norepinephrine. However, just as there are two types of cholinergic receptors, so too are there two types of adrenergic receptors. This section deals with the pharmacology of the adrenergic transmitter and some of the various agents that affect the activity of the two types of adrenergic receptors.

Interference with the Synthesis of Norepinephrine

Although it is well established that the amino acid *l*-tyrosine is taken up by adrenergic neurons for the production of norepinephrine, no specific drugs have as yet been synthesized for purposes of interfering with this uptake mechanism. Howover, it is possible to affect the levels of norepinephrine in adrenergic nerves by blocking the conversion of tyrosine to dopa, one of the precursors of norepinephrine. This conversion step can be blocked quite readily by administering the compound α-methyl-*p*-tyrosine. This compound acts to inhibit the activity of the enzyme tyrosine hydroxylase, which catalyzes the synthesis of dopa from tyrosine. The next stage in the formation of norepinephrine involves the conversion of dopa to dopamine, a reaction that is catalyzed by the enzyme dopa decarboxylase. The activity of this enzyme can be inhibited by either α-methyl-*m*-tyrosine or α-methyldopa. However, these substances do not inhibit the synthesis of norepinephrine. Instead, they act to lower tissue levels of norepinephrine by a process involving the production of a "false adrenergic transmitter" (see below). The final step in the formation of the transmitter involves the conversion of dopamine to norepinephrine by the enzyme dopamine-β-hydroxylase. Disulfiram (Antabuse) is sometimes administered to experimental subjects for purposes of inhibiting the activity of this particular enzyme. This results in a depletion of the tissue levels of norepinephrine but not dopamine in adrenergic neurons. A summary of these enzymes and the substances used to inhibit their activity is presented in Table 5.4. Of the three important enzymes mentioned above, only tyrosine hydroxylase is present in rather low concentrations relative to its substrate, tyrosine. The other two enzymes, dopa decarboxylase and dopamine-β-hydroxylase, on the other hand, are present in much greater concentrations relative to their respective substrates, dopa and dopamine. This means that inhibition of these enzymes has relatively minor effects on the overall levels of nor-epinephrine in adrenergic tissue unless inhibition of their activity is complete. Inhibition of tyrosine hydroxylase, however, produces a significant depletion of norepinephrine levels owing to its low concentration relative to its substrate. It is for this reason that the activity of this enzyme is spoken of as the "rate-limiting step" in the formation of norepinephrine.

Table 5.4   Enzymes and Enzyme Inhibitors of Various Steps in the Biosynthesis of Catecholamines

Enzyme	Inhibitor
Tyrosine hydroxylase	α-Methyl-p-tyrosine
Dopa decarboxylase	α-Methyldopa
	α-Methyl-m-tyrosine
Dopamine-β-hydroxylase	Disulfiram (Antabuse)

It should be apparent that the various drugs that are able to inhibit these particular enzymes are potentially valuable tools for investigating the role of dopamine and norepinephrine in behavior. For instance, if the investigator were interested in the behavioral effects of reducing all the catecholamines in the brain, he might consider using α-methyl-p-tyrosine. A more specific question might involve the role of norepinephrine, and this could be explored somewhat through the administration of disulfiram, which has the effect of lowering norepinephrine levels (and raising dop-amine levels).

Interference with the synthesis of norepinephrine may also be accom-plished in another manner which involves the formation of "false neuro-chemical transmitters." These false transmitters are substances that are capable of replacing norepinephrine and of being released from adrenergic terminals following stimulation of adrenergic neurons (see review by Kopin, 1972). But although they resemble norepinephrine in structure, they lack its sympathomimetic activity.

False transmitters can be introduced into adrenergic neurons because dopamine decarboxylase, the enzyme responsible for the conversion of dopa to dopamine, is not very specific in its activity. Thus substances which are similar in structure to dopa such as α-methyldopa and α-methyl-m-tyrosine are accepted as substrates and are transformed into α-methyl-dopamine and α-methyl-m-tyranine, respectively. These in turn are converted into the false neurotransmitters α-methylnorepinephrine (Cobefrine) and metaraminol, respectively. Since these false neurotransmitters are stored in adrenergic tissue, the neuronal levels of norepinephrine are lowered. Consequently, there is a concomitant decrease in the amount of active physiological transmitter to react with postsynaptic receptors following the propagation of an action potential in adrenergic neurons.

Interference with Storage

A number of drugs are able to produce fairly long lasting depletions of norepinephrine from its binding sites. The prototype of this class of compound is the rauwolfia alkaloid reserpine, although guanethidine can also be used for this purpose. The main difference between the two as far as locus of action is concerned, is that reserpine can penetrate the blood-brain barrier, whereas guanethidine cannot. Therefore, the latter compound has no direct CNS effects.

Both reserpine and guanethidine promote the release of catecholamines and serotonin from their storage sites and impair the binding of newly synthesized quantities of these biogenic amines. These amines are then exposed to immediate metabolic inactivation, and therefore they cannot be accumulated in sufficient quantity for subsequent adrenergic nerve transmission. The result is tantamount to a blockade of adrenergic receptors.

Like reserpine and quanethidine, tetrabenazine also causes depletion of norepinephrine from its binding sites, but whereas reserpine and guanethidine produce a long-lasting depletion, that promoted by tetrabenazine is relatively brief.

Still another group of drugs which are thought to exert their effects by depleting norepinephrine stores is the amphetamines. Although both reserpine and amphetamine deplete endogenous norepinephrine from its stores, each produces diametrically opposite behavioral effects. This is because reserpine causes a slow prolonged liberation of norepinephrine, which is then metabolized while still present in the vicinity of its storage sites and thus prior to its discharge into the synaptic cleft. In contrast, amphetamine promotes a relatively large, rapid, and brief depletion of norepinephrine which is not metabolized before it is able to react with its receptors. Consequently, whereas the norepinephrine stores depleted by reserpine lack physiological activity, those liberated by amphetamine produce a distinct sympathomimetic effect.

The actual destruction of adrenergic nerve terminals can now be accomplished by treatment with the compound 6-hydroxydopamine (see review by Thoenen, 1972). This substance has the effect of depleting norepinephrine from adrenergic tissues for long periods, resulting in what is sometimes referred to as "chemical sympathectomy." If administered to adult animals, these effects are not permanent. On the other hand, if given to very young animals, the chemical sympathectomy tends to be irreversible (Thoenen, 1971). This effect, however, is confined to peripheral adrenergic neurons since 6-hydroxydopamine does not pass through the blood barrier (cf. Laverty et al., 1965; Porter et al., 1963). To explore its central effects, it must be injected directly into the brain.

Inhibition of Uptake Mechanisms

It has already been noted that once norepinephrine has reacted with its receptors it is taken back into presynaptic adrenergic terminals by an "amine pump". Since this mechanism constitutes an important source for the replenishment of norepinephrine in adrenergic tissue, drugs such as imipramine, amitriptyline and desipramine which inhibit its activity are able to deplete markedly tissue levels of norepinephrine. The mechanism of action of these compounds is believed to involve their competition with norepinephrine for the sites on the amine pump which carry it back into adrenergic tissue. As a result, there is less of the physiological transmitter available for reacting with postsynaptic receptors following an action potential. The effect of these drugs is thus similar to that resulting from depletion of norepinephrine levels by reserpine and guanethidine, or that resulting from the replacement of norepinephrine by false neurochemical transmitters.

Interference with Release

Another aspect of the effects of bretylium, guanethidine, and the local anaesthetic lidocaine (xylocholine) is that they have the ability to block the release of norepinephrine from adrenergic tissue by some mechanism which is still not understood. However, this activity is confined mainly to the peripheral nervous system since these compounds do not penetrate the blood-brain barrier readily.

In dealing with the release of norepinephrine from its stores, attention should be drawn briefly to the Burn-Rand (1962) hypothesis. As noted previously (p. 30), this hypothesis argues that acetylcholine acts to bring about the release of norepinephrine from synaptic vesicles. Experimental verification for this hypothesis, as far as the central nervous system is involved, has been provided by Philippu (1970), who showed that acetylcholine promotes the release of catecholamines from the hypothalamus. A detailed survey reviewing the effects of cholinomimetic drugs on the release of catecholamines can be found in Muscholl (1970).

Stimulation of Receptors

Just as there are two basic cholinergic receptors, there are also two main adrenergic receptors; these have been designated as α and β by Ahlquist (1948). Ahlquist's classification is based on the responses to six different sympathomimetic amines of a number of peripheral organs such as the isolated cardiac and smooth muscle preparations taken from several different species. For the α receptors, norepinephrine was one of the most, and isoproterenol one of the least, potent sympathomimetics. Those at which isoproterenol was the most, and norepinephrine the least, potent were labeled β receptors.

As a result of the acceptance of Ahlquist's demonstration, it is now rather commonplace to refer to sympathomimetic agents and adrenoreceptor blocking compounds in terms of their specific receptor activity. Some of the blocking compounds are in fact so selective in their activity that they are often used to identify the kind of receptor for a certain drug on the basis of whether or not the actions of the drug in question are attenuated by prior administration of the blocking compound.

The most widely used sympathomimetic amines are phenylephrine, norepinephrine, epinephrine, isoproterenol, ephedrine, and amphetamine. The first three of these compounds elicit their effects by acting directly on postsynaptic α-adrenergic receptors. The third compound also acts directly on adrenergic receptors, but those receptors are predominantly of the β type. In general it appears that stimulation of α receptors has an excitatory effect on behavior, whereas stimulation of β receptors tends to depress ongoing behavior. The remaining two substances, ephedrine and amphetamine, act indirectly by causing the release of norepinephrine from its storage sites, but it is also possible that they have some direct stimulating effects on both α and β receptors as well (cf. Mennear and Rudzik, 1965).

Adrenergic Blocking Compounds

Drugs that antagonize responses elicited by sympathomimetic amines are sometimes referred to as adrenolytics or sympatholytics.

α-ADRENERGIC BLOCKING DRUGS

Two of the most widely used drugs of this type are dibenamine and phenoxydibenzamine. Because the blocking actions of these two agents last for several weeks, they are classified as "irreversible" blockers. In contrast, the α blockers, azapetine, phentolamine, piperoxan, and tolazoline, and considered "reversible" blockers since their half-life is only about 24 hours following a single injection. However, their effects can still be detected for 3 to 4 days after administration; should administration be repeated on a daily basis, the effects tend to be cumulative. The ergot alkaloids, ergotamine and dihydroergotamine, should also be mentioned at this point since they too are potent α-blocking agents.

β-ADRENERGIC BLOCKING DRUGS

The most potent drug in this class is propranolol. Dichloroisoproterenol (DCI) and pronethanol are also potent β blockers, but one of the difficulties in evaluating the effects of these substances is that they tend to have major side effects not related to their blocking action.

Interference with the Inactivation of Norepinephrine

Although monoamine oxidase (MAO) and catechol-O-methyl transferase (COMT) account for only part of the process involved in the termination of catecholamine effects in the CNS, inhibition of these substances, especially MAO, has marked behavioral effects that are primarily excitatory. The MAO inhibitors are characterized by their capacity to inhibit the oxidative deamination of dopamine, norepinephrine, and serotonin. In addition, they potentiate and prolong the effects of those drugs which act by causing the release of these biogenic amines from their storage sites. However, drugs which are classified as MAO inhibitors also inhibit the activity of various other enzymes in the body, and consequently, behavioral effects produced by this class of compounds must be interpreted with caution. Currently, the main MAO inhibitors being used for experimental and/or clinical purposes are pargyline, nialamide, tranylcypromine, and isocarboxazid.

Table 5.5 provides a summary of compounds acting at the adrenergic synapse.

HUNGER: AN ADRENERGIC MECHANISM

Lesions in the medial part of the hypothalamus, especially the ventromedial nucleus, produce hyperphagia, whereas lesions in the lateral area

Table 5.5 Summary of Compounds Acting at the Adrenergic Synapse

Mechanism of Action	Compound	Effect
Interference with synthesis of NE		
Inhibition of rate-limiting enzyme	α-Methyl-p-tyrosine	Antiadrenergic
Production of "false transmitters"	α-Methyl-dopa, α-methyl-m-tyrosine	Antiadrenergic
Interference with uptake	Imipramine, amitriptyline	Antiadrenergic
Interference with storage	Reserpine, tetrabenazine, 6-hydroxydopamine	Antiadrenergic
Interference with release	Bretylium, guanethidine, iproniazid	Antiadrenergic
Promotion of release	Ephedrine, amphetamine, tyramine	Sympathomimetic
Stimulation of postsynaptic receptors		
α	Phenylephrine	Sympathomimetic
β	Isoproterenol	Sympathomimetic
Blockade of postsynaptic receptors		
α	Phenoxydibenzamine, phentolamine	Antiadrenergic
β	Propranolol	Antiadrenergic
Interference with enzymatic inactivation	Pargyline, tranylcypromine	Sympathomimetic

of the hypothalamus result in aphagia. The reverse of these effects can be produced by electrical stimulation of these areas. Thus electrical stimulation of the ventromedial hypothalamus inhibits feeding whereas electrical stimulation of the lateral hypothalamus induces feeding behavior. These observations have prompted the hypothesis that the hypothalamus contains a "stop-go" mechanism for the regulation of food intake, the ventromedial nucleus being the stop mechanism or satiety center and the lateral hypothalamus, the feeding center.

The lateral hypothalamus, it may be remembered, is also an area from which drinking can be elicited following the administration of cholinomimetic compounds. If adrenergic compounds are injected into the lateral hypothalamus, however, feeding behavior can be induced. Results such as these suggest that biological activities such as hunger and thirst are represented by parallel systems of neurons which pass through the hypothalamus

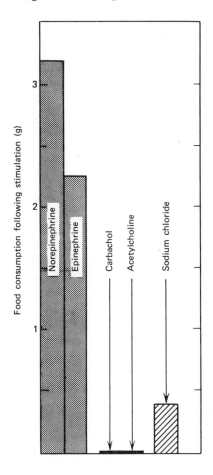

Fig. 5.5 Food intake during 1 hour following adrenergic stimulation of the lateral hypothalamus in satiated rats. Injections of both epinephrine and norepinephrine stimulated food intake around 5 to 10 minutes after administration, and this effect lasted for 20 to 40 minutes. Norepinephrine had a much greater effect on feeding than did epinephrine (from Grossman, 1960).

and which can be differentiated from one another on the basis of the neurochemicals liberated at their respective synapses. In this section, some of the pharmacological approaches that have been taken to elucidate the nature of the adrenergic mechanisms which mediate food intake are presented.

Figure 5.5 shows that the administration of the adrenergic compounds norepinephrine and epinephrine both elicit feeding behavior in satiated rats, whereas the cholinergic agents acetylcholine and carbachol are without effect on food intake.

Table 5.6 shows that this effect is mediated by α-adrenergic receptors since norepinephrine elicits feeding whereas the β-adrenergic stimulant isoproterenol does not.

Table 5.6 Effects of Adrenergic Stimulation of Lateral Hypothalamus on Food Intake in Satiated Rats[a]

Compound	Dose (μm moles)	Food Intake per Hour (g)
Norepinephrine	20	3.6
Isoproterenol	10	0.2
	40	0.3
	80	0.4
	150	0.9

[a] Modified from Slanger and Miller (1969).

Further evidence that feeding is mediated exclusively by α-adrenergic receptors is demonstrated by the fact that preadministration of the α-adrenergic blocking compound phentolamine is able to block norepinephrine induced feeding, whereas preadministration of the β-adrenergic blocking compound propranolol is without effect (see Table 5.7).

Table 5.7 Effects of Adrenergic Blocking Drugs on Norepinephrine (NE) (20 mμ moles) Induced Feeding[a]

Compound	Dose (mμ moles)	Food Intake per Hour (g)
Saline	—	4.0
Phentolamine	40	0.2
Propranolol	120	4.0

[a] Modified from Slanger and Miller (1969).

The effect of the α-adrenergic blocking compound dibenzyline on food intake following food deprivation is shown in Figure 5.6. It is apparent from the figure that this blocking compound does attenuate food intake but that the attenuation is not complete.

The effects of inhibition of monoamine oxidase with nialamide and/or the interference with storage of norepinephrine in synaptic terminals by tetrabenazine are shown in Table 5.8. Inspection of the table indicates that the combination of both these treatments has an effect roughly equal to that of norepinephrine applied directly to the same site. Supposedly, the effect of the monoamine oxidase inhibitor is that of preventing the breakdown of norepinephrine in the synaptic terminal, whereas the effect of tetrabenazine is that of preventing the binding of norepinephrine in synaptic vesicles. As a result, an excess of norepinephrine builds up in the pre-

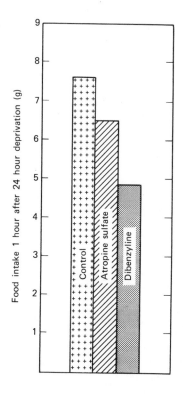

Fig. 5.6 Food intake of 24-hour food-deprived animals 1 hour after central application of adrenergic (dibenzyline) or cholinergic (atropine) blocking agents. Although atropine tended to suppress eating, the extent of the suppression was significantly greater with dibenzyline. Control levels represent food intake of 24-hour deprived rats without blocking agents (from Grossman, 1962b).

Table 5.8 Effects of Nialamide and Tetrabenazine on Norepinephrine Induced Feeding in Satiated Rats[a]

Compound	Dose (mμ moles)	Food Intake per Hour (g)
Norepinephrine	20	3.5
Tetrabenazine	100	0.6
+ nialamide	200	0.7
Nialamide	200	1.0
+ tetrabenazine	100	2.9

[a] Modified from Slanger and Miller (1969).

synaptic terminals and then spills out into the synapse, thus coming into contact with the receptors mediating food intake.

However, this effect on food intake is not simply the result of norepinephrine causing the stimulation of effector mechanisms involved in food intake. Evidence that this is not the case is presented in Figure 5.7, which

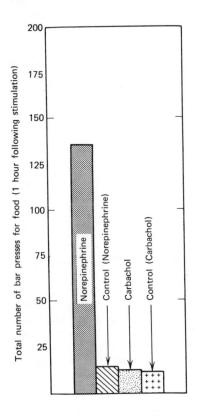

Fig. 5.7 Effects of adrenergic stimulation of the lateral hypothalamus of satiated rats on the rate of bar pressing for food reward. Control levels were determined during a 1-hour period preceding each stimulation (from Grossman, 1962a).

shows that centrally applied norepinephrine is able to induce bar pressing for food reward.

Although norepinephrine-induced feeding does in many ways resemble the kind of behavior that can be produced by food deprivation, there are certain anomalies which make the parallel between the two still rather hypothetical. For one thing, chemically induced feeding is unable to maintain operant responding on certain schedules, although such responding is maintained with food deprivation (Coons and Quartermain, 1970). Secondly, norepinephrine induced feeding is influenced by small changes in the palatability of available food to a much greater extent than that which is observed following food deprivation (Booth and Quartermain, 1965). Finally, adrenergic blocking compounds are unable to attenuate feeding following food deprivation to the same extent as that which occurs in connection with norepinephrine induced food intake. Consequently, it must be concluded that although feeding behavior may involve α-adrenergic pathways, other factors contributing to "hunger" involve nonadrenergic mechanisms.

PHARMACOLOGY OF SEROTONERGIC MECHANISMS

In general, there has been a minimal amount of work devoted to the behavioral pharmacology of serotonergic mechanisms since serotonin's role as a neurotransmitter is even more conjectural than those of acetylcholine and norepinephrine. Furthermore, many of the compounds that affect the activity of adrenergically mediated synapses also tend to affect those mediated by serotonin. Consequently, a discussion of these compounds such as that presented in the preceding section would be repetitious.

This does not mean that there are no specific drugs affecting the serotonergic system. For instance, the drug p-chlorophenylalanine (pCPA) is quite selective in reducing tissue levels of serotonin. This reduction occurs via the inhibition of tryptophan 5-hydroxylase, the enzyme which converts dietary tryptophan to 5-hydroxytryptophan, the immediate precursor of serotonin.

There are also several chemicals which antagonize the effects of serotonin. Among these is the well-known hallucinogen lysergic acid diethylamide (LSD). A compound with similar action but no hallucinatory effect is 2-bromolysergic acid diethylamide (BOL). Two other potent antagonists of the actions of serotonin are methylsergide and cyproheptadine.

The main enzyme which inactivates serotonin is MAO. Therefore, the list of drugs that was mentioned with respect to the inhibition of MAO in the section dealing with the pharmacology of norepinephrine is also pertinent to serotonin.

SEXUAL BEHAVIOR AND SEROTONERGIC MECHANISMS

Although the involvement of the male and female hormones in the maintenance of sexual behavior has long been recognized, it is only recently that the relationship between cerebral neurochemicals and sexual behavior has been investigated. One of the more interesting features of this problem is the apparent relationship between this aspect of behavior and 5-hydroxytryptamine in both male and female animals (e.g., Gawienowski and Hodgen, 1971; Gessa et al., 1970; and Myerson, 1964). For example, whereas pargyline causes a significant decrease in the heterosexual behavior of male rats (see Table 5.9), pCPA, which selectively depletes cerebral 5-HT, not only reverses this effect but also induces compulsive sexual activity in male animals of several species, including rats, cats, and rabbits (Tagliamonte et al., 1967, 1970; Ferguson et al., 1970). That this effect is due to the action of these drugs on 5-HT rather than on the other amines in the CNS is evident from an inspection of Table 5.9. The data presented in this table indicate that sexual behavior is inhibited following treatment with pargyline but is increased following pCPA.

Table 5.9. Effects of Pargyline and/or pCPA on Sexual Behavior and Brain Amine Content of Male Rats (μg/g)[a]

Treatment	N	Rats Copulating (%)	5-HT	NE	DA
None	30	63	0.50	0.48	0.80
Paragyline	30	10	1.20	0.68	1.16
pCPA + pargyline	30	100	0.03	0.40	0.75
pCPA	30	100	0.08	0.58	0.83

[a] Adapted from Tagliamonte et al., 1971.

This relationship between 5-HT and sexual behavior has led to the assumption that 5-HT pathways exert an inhibitory influence over sexual behavior. The nature of this inhibition appears to involve the antagonistic interaction between 5-HT and testosterone in male rats since castration abolishes the compulsive sexual behavior produced by pCPA, whereas testosterone potentiates it (see Table 5.10).

Table 5.10 Effects of Castration and Testosterone on the Sexual Behavior of Male Rats Treated with *p*-Chlorophenylalanine[a]

Treatment	Rats Exhibiting Mounting (%)	
	Intact	Castrated
pCPA	27.5	0
pCPA + testosterone	100	80
Testosterone	12.5	0

[a] Modified from Gessa et al. (1970).

The compulsive nature of the effects of decreased serotonin levels on sexual behavior is evident from the fact that not only is heterosexual behavior increased by the administration of pCPA, but homosexual behavior between male rats is also increased (see Table 5.11). However, it is not known as yet whether these effects are produced as a result of an increase in general motivation, or because of some direct effect on the effector mechanisms involved in sexual behavior.

Table 5.11 Homosexual Behavior in Male Rats Following Treatment with p-Chlorophenylalanine[a]

Treatment	N	Median Number of Mounts	Median Number of Seminal Emissions
Control	5	0	0
pCPA + pargyline	5	24	4

[a] Modified from Gawienowski and Hodgen (1971).

PSYCHOPHARMACOLOGICAL AGENTS

During the last 25 years a dramatic change in the psychiatric treatment of behavioral disorders has occurred, a change marked by the increasing use of chemical agents. Administration of these compounds has done more for the rapid discharge of patients from hospitals than has any other method of therapy, and there are no signs of a diminution in the use of drugs in this regard.

Surprisingly, however, most of the discoveries of the behavioral effects of these drugs have come not from the laboratory, but from observations of patients who were given these agents initially for purposes other than their behavioral disorders. It was only after these drugs were found to be useful in the treatment of various behavioral disorders that research programs were begun in which animals rather than humans were used to try to discover the actual sites and modes of action of these behaviorally active compounds. However, despite the fact that most of the discoveries in psychopharmacology have had their origins in the clinic rather than in the laboratory, it is only under the controlled environmental conditions of the laboratory that a rational scientific basis has been elucidated for the continued use of these drugs. A thorough understanding of where and how a drug acts, after all, is essential if new, therapeutically more useful drugs are to be developed.

As noted at the outset of this chapter, the problem of selecting acceptable criteria for the placement of drugs into meaningful categories has yet to be solved to everyone's satisfaction. Despite wide disagreement concerning classification among various disciplines, psychoactive drugs have been dichotomized into two main functional groups—CNS depressants and CNS stimulants. These two groups of drugs have been subclassed further on the basis of their sites and mechanisms of action. The general outlines of this tentative classification are followed for purposes of discussion. The material covered in the remainder of this chapter is representative of the majority of psychoactive drugs currently in therapeutic or experimental use; in no way should it be viewed as a survey of the literature. The intent is merely to provide an orientation for further study. Those interested in greater detail and/or scope should consult any of the standard references in pharmacology such as Goodman and Gilman (1970), DiPalma (1971), or Aviado (1972).

CNS DEPRESSANTS

Depressant drugs are so-called because they reduce the excitability of nervous tissue in the brain. Although depressant drugs are generally separated into different categories such as anesthetics and hypnotics, the mechanism of action of all the depressant drugs is thought to be basically that of depositing themselves in bulk in cell membranes because of their affinity for lipoid matter. Although the details of their action are still uncertain, it is possible that their presence in the cell membrane acts to produce enzymatic changes in membrane activity leading to a diminution of cellular metabolism which is reflected in reduced excitability. The various drugs that act in this manner, however, seem to affect some areas of the brain before others, and they have been classified subsequently in terms of their therapeutic applications.

GENERAL ANESTHETICS

The term anesthesia means "without sensation." In other words, anesthesia is a condition in which the subject cannot perceive sensory stimuli, especially pain. The general class of drugs which are used to produce this particular effect is called anesthetics; typically these are dichotomized into those that are volatile and those that are nonvolatile. The volatile anesthetics, for example, ethyl ether, chloroform, and halothane, are all administered by inhalation and tend to block pain as well as all the other sensory pathways as the dosage is increased. The nonvolatile anesthetics such as the short-acting barbiturates thiopental and hexobarbital are administered intravenously and they produce only a partial blockade of sensory nerve impulses.

Volatile Anesthetics

To facilitate discussion of the various effects produced by these drugs, it is customary to separate the phenomenon of anesthesia into four stages, each stage being related directly to the concentration of the compound in the central nervous system.

1. Analgesia. The first stage of anesthesia is called analgesia because there is a loss of sensation involving touch and pain.

2. Light Anesthesia. This stage of anesthesia is characterized by a loss of voluntary motor activity, increased reflex activity, and loss of "consciousness."

3. Surgical Anesthesia. This stage is marked by a diminution of muscle tone and abolition of spontaneous muscular activity. This is the level of anesthesia in which most surgical operations are conducted.

4. Medullary Paralysis. In this final stage of anesthesia, there is an inhibition of medullary function resulting in respiratory failure. Death results if this condition is maintained.

The volatile general anesthetics are taken up rapidly from the lungs. Distribution is dependent on blood flow and the solubility of these compounds in the various tissues of the body. Since these compounds have a high oil/water partition coefficient, they become concentrated for the most part in lipids. Thus, as a result of its rich blood supply and its relatively high lipid content, the brain is one of the first areas of the body to be affected.

For the most part, the volatile anesthetics are not metabolized to any great extent, but rather they leave the body essentially unchanged in the way they entered it—through the lungs. This begins to occur as a result of a change in the concentration gradient. Once the source of the gas has been removed, and the concentration of the anesthetic in the brain becomes greater than that in the blood, it begins to move into the blood and for the same reason, it moves out of the blood and into the lungs.

The cellular mechanism of action of these compounds appears to involve a depression of the nerve cell membrane's potential excitability. For example, as a result of their affinity for the lipoprotein material in the cell membrane, the general anesthetics tend to move into this part of the cell. In so doing, they saturate the cell membrane and interfere thereby with the permeability of the membrane to the ions whose movements account for the neuronal action potential. The main site of action appears to be the nonspecific reticular activating system and the thalamic relays. The decrease in the excitability of these systems more than likely accounts for the onset of the early stages of anesthesia.

In addition to their enormous benefit to surgery, some of the general anesthetics are now beginning to find their way into psychopharmacology as well. For instance, both nitrous oxide and carbon dioxide have been shown to have a beneficial effect in the treatment of certain kinds of neurotic disorders. Wolpe (1958) has suggested that although the direct anxiety-reducing effects of gases such as carbon dioxide are only temporary, they do facilitate treatment by techniques which eventually do lead to permanent cures. In his own case, Wolpe employs the method of "reciprocal inhibition" in which he teaches his patients to make a response which inhibits anxiety during exposure to an anxiety-eliciting situation. As a result, the strength of the anxiety-provoking situation is reduced. The response most often used to inhibit anxiety is relaxation, the rationale being that it is impossible to be anxious if one is completely relaxed. Some patients are simply not capable of relaxing deeply enough for the procedure to work, however, and in such patients, carbon dioxide is administered to enable them to achieve the anxiety-free state long enough for the "reciprocal inhibition" process to occur.

Before passing on to the nonvolatile anesthetics, some mention should be made of a group of compounds which produce the same kinds of effects as the general anesthetics but which are used primarily as solvents in industry rather than for medical purposes. These compounds are the volatile aromatic hydrocarbons such as benzene, toluene, and xylene, which are found in paint thinners, lighter fluids, glue, etc. When their vapors are inhaled (sniffed), many of the symptoms of the first stage of general anesthesia, along with feelings of dizziness, exhilaration, visual hallucinations, etc., are produced. Prolonged administration, however, produces general depression of the CNS leading to the second stage of general anesthesia. These substances do not appear to have any addiction liability, but psychological dependence may develop in certain individuals as a result of their prolonged abuse of these materials.

Nonvolatile Anesthetics

Among the most frequently used of these drugs are thiopental (Pentothal), methohexital (Brevital), and hexobarbital. The main drawback of these agents is that their time course of action cannot be influenced as easily as that of the volatile anesthetics. Like the latter, however, their main effect is on the reticular activating system, the inhibitory components being affected before the excitatory, thus accounting for an initial stimulantlike effect followed by depression. However, unlike the volatile anesthetics, the primary sensory pathways remain relatively unaffected at therapeutic doses so that the subject is able to receive sensory input.

Because these drugs do not inhibit sensory impulses, they are used rarely in surgery except as an adjunct to anesthesia with the volatile gases. On the other hand, thiopental has recently been used successfully in the treatment of anxiety phobias. In the course of such treatment, the patient receives an intravenous injection of either pentothal or Brevital at a dose sufficient enough to induce sleep. Since these drugs are rapidly excreted, their effects usually last for only about 15 to 30 minutes. According to the results of one study comparing this treatment with placebo injections, after 3 months 85% of the drug-treated group had improved compared with only a 50% improvement rate for the placebo-injected patients (King and Little, 1959).

In contrast to Pentothal and Brevital, the third nonvolatile anesthetic, hexobarbital, is used primarily in laboratory experiments for purposes of inducing the loss of the "righting reflex" in animals. This rather easily produced effect can then be used as a dependent variable in measuring tolerance and cross-tolerance to hexobarbital and to other compounds, respectively.

LOCAL ANESTHETICS

Like the general anesthetics, the group of drugs known as the local anesthetics, for example, procaine, lidocaine, and cocaine, depress the excitability of nerve cells. However, in contrast to the general anesthetics, these drugs are usually applied topically to certain areas in order to block pain sensation.

The mechanism by which the local anesthetics block conduction is through their interference with the influx of sodium ions during depolarization and their interference with the efflux of potassium ions during repolarization, both of which are fundamental to the generation of the action potential. Although they do not depolarize or hyperpolarize the resting membrane potential themselves, the local anesthetics raise the threshold for the initiation of impulses, decrease the amplitude, and reduce the velocity of conduction of action potentials. The exact way in which this is accomplished is still unknown, but it has been suggested that they dissolve in the cell membrane and thereby narrow the size of the pores through which sodium ions flow. Alternatively, it has been proposed that the local anesthetics increase the surface pressure at the level of the cell membrane and the extracellular fluid, and that this pressure causes a narrowing of the pores through which sodium ions enter the cell.

The local anesthetics act on the smaller pain fibers in the peripheral nervous system prior to affecting the larger sensory and motor neurons. Consequently, if the concentration of the local anesthetic is kept to a minimum there is usually little impairment of other sensory or motor activity. To further minimize the chances of undesirable effects, the local anesthetics usually are administered in conjunction with epinephrine. The latter causes vasoconstriction of blood vessels, thus curtailing the flow of blood to the area treated by the anesthetic. Consequently, the possibility of the drug entering the general circulation from its site of application is reduced.

Although cocaine was once a widely used local anesthetic around the turn of the century, it was replaced quickly by the newer synthetic agents such as procaine because of the CNS excitatory effect of cocaine.

At low doses, some of the effects of cocaine are exhilaration, increased motor activity, and a feeling of increased capacity for physical work. Indeed, the leaves of the cocoa plant, from which cocaine is derived, have long been chewed by the natives of Peru and Bolivia to increase their physical endurance and to give them a sense of well-being. It is for the inducement of such feelings that cocaine has become a main drug of abuse in this country.

It is believed that the excitatory effects of this drug are due to its depression of inhibitory centers in the cortex. As the dosage is increased, however, depression of the excitatory centers also begins to occur. At the level of the medulla, the respiratory centers are likewise initially stimulated and then depressed. With very large doses, however, respiration is completely depressed and death occurs.

SEDATIVE-HYPNOTICS

Sedatives are drugs that supposedly depress nervous activity without producing sleep. Hypnotics produce both depression of nervous activity and sleep. However, the distinction between these two classes of drugs is not really very meaningful, since in large doses sedatives also produce sleep, and on the other hand, sleep is not necessarily induced by the hypnotics in low doses. Moreover, at very high doses, both produce anesthesia. The principal medical uses for these drugs is to reduce anxiety ("tranquilize") and/or to induce sleep. The depressant effect is similar to that produced by alcohol and is characterized by drowsiness, euphoria, uncoordinated movement, slurred speech, and impaired thinking and memory.

Some of the oldest of the drugs that have been used to produce relaxation of the sedative-hypnotic variety are sodium and potassium bromide, chloral hydrate, and paraldehyde. The "Mickey Finn" that was used to sedate sailors so that they could be "shanghaied" aboard undesirable sailing vessels was actually a mixture of chloral hydrate and alcohol. None of these compounds is used widely at present, however, because of undesirable side effects associated with each of them. Instead, the most commonly encountered group of sedative-hypnotic drugs today is the barbiturates.

The barbiturates are all derivatives of barbituric acid which, oddly enough, has no sedative-hypnotic activity of its own. In small doses, the barbiturates tend to relieve anxiety without necessarily inducing sleep. On the contrary, there may even be a feeling of euphoria and excitement produced by low doses of these drugs. Individuals suffering from anxiety seem especially prone to misuse of these drugs for just this purpose.

The antianxiety effects of the barbiturates have in fact been demonstrated repeatedly in the laboratory in animals suffering from "experimental neuroses" (Masserman, 1962). The general experimental procedure used by Masserman involves first training an animal such as a cat to press a lever in order to receive food. Once this has been learned, the animal is given a blast of air or an electric shock whenever it continues to press the bar, thus creating a conflict situation—if the animal wishes to allay his hunger, he must be willing to accept pain. After being in this state of conflict for a while, nearly all animals exhibit "deviations in behavior sufficiently marked, generalized and persistent to be termed experimental neuroses" (Masserman, 1962), for example, fast heartbeat, disorganization of learned skills, gastrointestinal dysfunctioning, compulsive stereotyped behavior, loss of social dominance in a group, and sexual deviations such as homosexuality or autoeroticism. When treated with barbiturates, however, these animals exhibit marked improvements which are much greater than those produced by drugs such as alcohol, reserpine, chlorpromazine, or meprobamate (see below).

The sense of euphoria produced by low doses of these drugs is generally thought to occur as a result of an initial release of the inhibitory control exercised by the cortex over the reticular formation. If the dosage is increased, however, the excitatory effects on the reticular formation are also diminished and sedation begins to occur. Barbiturate-induced sleep is different from normal sleep, however, in that it curtails the frequency of rapid eye movements (REM) indicative of dreaming episodes. As the individual continues to take these drugs, however, the amount of REM sleep per night gradually returns to normal, apparently as a result of the development of tolerance to this effect. On the other hand, should use of the drug be discontinued, there is often a "rebound" increase in REM sleep for several nights, apparently making up for what was lost during the initial period of drug administration. In some cases, this extra REM sleep is often associated with the experience of "nightmares" and sensations of not having slept well (Oswald and Priest, 1965). This effect on the sleep cycle may thus reflect the development of tolerance and physical dependence commonly found in many physiologically addicting drugs.

If the dosage is increased above that necessary to overcome insomnia, the activity of the reticular formation eventually becomes completely blocked and a state of general anesthesia ensues. If the dosage is increased still further, there is a progressive loss of reflex activity and depression of respiratory and vasomotor functions due to the action of these drugs on these centers in the medulla, and finally death results.

At present, more than 2000 kinds of barbiturates have been synthesized, many of which have been tested pharmacologically and marketed. On the basis of their onsets and durations of action, these barbiturates frequently are differentiated into one of four classes:

1. Ultrashort-acting (less than 1 hour), for example, thiopental.
2. Short-acting (less than 3 hours), for example, pentobarbital.
3. Intermediate-acting (3 to 6 hours), for example, amobarbital.
4. Long-acting (more than 6 hours), for example, phenobarbital.

However, this distinction is somewhat arbitrary since both the onset and the duration of action of these drugs varies as a function of dosage and route of administration.

In general, the barbiturate drugs are absorbed well from both oral and parenteral injection sites. The partition coefficients and pK_a values of some of the more common barbiturates are shown in Table 5.12. Inspection of the table indicates that the high oil/water coefficient of thiopental would result in its being rapidly absorbed across various cell membranes including the blood-brain barrier, thus accounting for its ultrashort onset of activity.

Table 5.12   Physicochemical Characteristics of Some Common Barbiturates

Barbiturate	Trade Name	Oil/Water Partition Coefficient	pK_a
Barbital	Veronal	1	7.8
Phenobarbital	Luminal	3	7.3
Pentobarbital	Nembutal	39	8.0
Secobarbital	Seconal	52	7.9
Thiopental	Pentothal	580	7.4

Although the behavioral effects of the barbiturates cannot be attributed to any single specific action at the cellular level, one effect which does seem to be common to many of these drugs is an interference with the mechanism of oxidative phosphorylation in the CNS (see p. 8). This conclusion is based on the observation that the barbiturates decrease the concentration of inorganic phosphates and with it the utilization of ATP in the CNS, as indicated by a diminished uptake of oxygen by the brain. In addition, it has also been demonstrated that the barbiturates decrease oxidative metabolism in cellular mitochondria.

Metabolism of most of the barbiturates occurs primarily in the liver, which changes these drugs into metabolites that are more polar than the parent compounds. These metabolites are then removed from the blood mainly by the kidney.

The phenomenon of tolerance tends to develop rather rapidly to most of the effects of the barbiturates. The mechanism of this tolerance development mainly involves an increase in the activity of the enzymes of the liver which are responsible for their metabolism. This results in a faster rate of inactivation which is manifested by a decrease in magnitude of effect. As a consequence, more drug has to be taken in order to produce the effect obtained when the drug was first taken. However, tolerance does not develop to the toxicity associated with high doses of barbiturates. This means that as the dosage is increased to obtain sleep, the user approaches closer and closer to a dose that will be lethal. This cause of death is in fact common. In the United States, for example, barbiturate poisoning accounts for more deaths than any other kind of poisoning (Maynert, 1971). Barbiturate poisoning is not always accidental, however. Suicide by barbiturate poisoning, for example, rose from 0.9% in 1942 to 13.5% in 1962 for males and from 1.0 to 27.6% for females during this same time period (Shepherd et al., 1968).

In addition to producing tolerance, chronic use of barbiturates also results in physical addiction; the incidence of such addiction is in fact greater than addiction to narcotic drugs such as heroin (Maynert, 1971).

The severity of the withdrawal effects varies with the degree of previous usage. Following chronic use of high doses, abrupt withdrawal often results in convulsions, nausea, insomnia, delerium, and weight loss. The severity of this abstinence syndrome often is considered to be more dangerous than that associated with withdrawal from narcotic drugs. As a result of the aversiveness of such an experience, the barbiturate addict often continues to use his drug so as to avoid precipitating these withdrawal symptoms in himself.

ALCOHOL

The term alcohol generally refers to ethyl alcohol, the primary active ingredient in many fermented beverages. Until the middle of the 1800s, ethyl alcohol was a widely used general anesthetic because of its depressant effects on the CNS. However, with the introduction of chloroform and ether, its use in this regard was diminished by these newer and more efficacious agents. Today ethyl alcohol is used mainly for its intoxicant effects.

The main pharmacological site of action is the central nervous system, where its effects are somewhat related to those produced by the barbiturates. In fact, cross-tolerance between these two classes of agents has been observed, and this suggests that there may be some mechanism of action common to both.

As with most drugs, the effects of ethyl alcohol on behavior are related closely to its concentration in the body. At low doses, alcohol has relatively minor behavioral effects which are characterized by a sense of euphoria and stimulation. This sensation is one of the reasons alcohol is regarded incorrectly as a stimulant by many people. The reason for this initial reaction is that in its actions on the CNS, alcohol first affects the inhibitory centers of the cortex and by disrupting their functioning, it releases the excitatory centers from inhibition (disinhibition). The nature of the behavioral effect when this occurs, however, depends on the individual's prior history. If he is someone who normally inhibits his feelings toward others, these feelings may now be exhibited since his inhibitions have been suppressed. As the dosage is increased, however, there is a progressive deterioration of function beginning with a disruption of intellectual functioning, followed by an impairment of motor coordination, loss of consciousness, anesthesia, respiratory depression, and heart failure. These effects correspond to the progressive effects of the compound on the cortex, cerebellum, and medulla.

Alcohol is absorbed rapidly from the gastrointestinal tract by simple diffusion. Distribution is also fairly rapid. The well endowed blood supply of the brain coupled with its high lipid content account for the fact that the CNS is one area of the body most readily affected by this substance. Metabolism by the liver accounts for nearly all of the inactivation of this compound. Any alcohol that escapes metabolism is excreted mainly through the kidneys and the lungs. However, excessive intake of alcohol does produce an aftereffect, even though it is no longer present in the body. This aftereffect is the well-known "hangover" syndrome, which is characterized by a throbbing headache, tremors, dizziness, weakness, nausea, and vomiting. These effects are more common with the use of alcohol than with any of the other sedative-hypnotic drugs.

Tolerance to many of the behavioral effects of this substance has long been recognized, and as noted above, cross-tolerance between alcohol and the barbiturate drugs has been reported (Fischer and Olsner, 1960). This may account for the resistance on the part of many alcoholics to the effects of this latter group of drugs. However, as with the barbiturates, so too with alcohol, tolerance to the more profound effects following the ingestion of large amounts of this substance does not occur. Similarly, as with the barbiturates, withdrawal from the chronic use of alcohol is considered to be much more dangerous to life than is withdrawal from narcotic drugs such as heroin.

MAJOR AND MINOR TRANQUILIZERS

These drugs resemble the sedative-hypnotics in many of their actions, but in general they are less hypnotic than the latter. For instance, in large doses they do not produce anesthesia. In addition they tend to be more selective in relieving anxiety, and they are also less likely to produce either psychological or physical dependence. Tranquilizing drugs are dichotomized into either major or minor tranquilizers. Another commonly used dichotomy for these drugs is that of antineurotic and antipsychotic agents, which describes their effects in more functional terms. The principal differences between these two subclasses as follows. (1) The major tranquilizers (antipsychotic agents) are used to treat psychotic disorders such as schizophrenia and manic-depression, which are characterized by dramatic alterations in behavior and experiences of delusions and hallucinations. Minor tranquilizers (antineurotic agents), by contrast, are useful only in treating behavioral disorders considered to be neurotic, for example, anxiety, phobias, and obsessive-compulsive behavior. Minor tranquilizers are not very effective in treating psychoses, and likewise the major tranquilizers are not very effective in treating neurotic disorders. (2) Major tranquilizers depress the activity of lower brain centers such as the medullary chemoreceptor trigger zone and the vomiting center; as a result they are used often to treat the nausea and vomiting associated with various disorders. Minor tranquilizers do not depress the activity of the lower brain centers and hence have little antiemetic effects. (3) The major tranquilizers produce distinctive extrapyramidal effects such as tremors and spasticity. In contrast, the minor tranquilizers tend to produce general muscular relaxation. (4) Major tranquilizers have a number of different effects on the autonomic nervous system. For instance, some of the phenothiazines (e.g., chlorpromazine) are potent α-adrenergic blocking agents. The minor tranquilizers, on the other hand, have very little autonomic activity. (5) Minor tranquilizers tend to have a biphasic effect on behavior which is dose dependent. For instance, with small doses, these drugs tend to produce a euphoric, excitatory state similar to that observed following small doses of alcohol or some of the barbiturates. With large doses, however, the effect is more one of sedation than excitement. By contrast, the effects of the major tranquilizers are monophasic. (6) Major tranquilizers are hardly ever abused, whereas this is often the case with the minor tranquilizers. (7) There is no development of tolerance following chronic use of the major tranquilizers. Tolerance can develop to the minor tranquilizers. (8) There is no withdrawal syndrome following abstinence from the major tranquilizers. Withdrawal symptoms can occur following abstinence from the minor tranquilizers. (9) Major tranquilizers suppress active avoidance behavior in animals at doses that do not also affect escape responding. At low doses minor tranquilizers have no effects on active avoidance or escape responding, whereas at high doses, they tend to suppress both avoidance and escape behavior. (10) Minor tranquilizers appear to attenuate the aversive effects of noxious stimuli in conflict situations. Major tranquilizers do not affect conflict behavior.

These basic differences are summarized in Table 5.13. The two subclasses will now be discussed in more detail.

Table 5.13   Comparison of Uses and Effects of Major and Minor Tranquilizers

Major Tranquilizers	Minor Tranquilizers
Used primarily for psychotic disorders	Used primarily for neurotic disorders
Depress general motor activity	Little effect on motor activity
Extrapyramidal effects (tremors)	No extrapyramidal effects
Autonomic effects	No autonomic effects
No psychological dependence	Psychological dependence
No tolerance	Tolerance
No withdrawal symptoms	Possible withdrawal effects
No anticonvulsive actions	Anticonvulsive activity
Suppress active avoidance behavior but not escape	Suppress both escape and active avoidance
No reduction of conflict	Reduce conflict behavior
Monophasic effects	Biphasic effects

Major Tranquilizers

The most important drugs falling into this subclass are derivatives of phenothiazine; the prototype of these is chlorpromazine (Thorazine). This drug originally was synthesized for its potential antihistaminic activity but clinical observations of its effects soon revealed it to possess an extraordinary ability to "tranquilize" the agitated behavior of previously unmanageable psychotics. With further testing, it has shown itself to be particularly effective in the treatment of psychotic behavior diagnosed as schizophrenia, of which there are several different subtypes. In "simple" schizophrenia, patients have lost contact with reality. For example, they often suffer from paranoid delusions in which they believe that others are "out to get them." As a result, their behavior often is quite unpredictable and characterized by violence and hostility. The catatonic schizophrenic, on the other hand, is one who remains immobile for prolonged periods of time during which he must be clothed and force-fed. However, this stuporous state may change rather unexpectedly to one of hyperexcitability and destructiveness. A third class of schizophrenia is characterized by rapid swings in behavior from maniacal to depressive activity.

In general, all these behavioral disturbances are characterized at some stage by hyperexcitability and agitation. Although the phenothiazines unquestionably cause sedation, the therapeutic value of these drugs in the treatment of psychotic disturbances is far superior to that produced by the sedative-hypnotic drugs such as the barbiturates. The difference between these two classes of drugs is especially evident in the conditioned avoidance testing situation.

As noted previously, this involves first training an animal to make some kind of response such as climbing a bar or jumping over a barrier when the floor of its cage is electrified. This is termed an escape response to an unconditioned stimulus (shock). The animal is then taught to make the same response to the sound of a buzzer warning him that the grids on the floor will soon be electrified. If he responds to the buzzer by jumping the barrier or climbing the pole before the shock, he is said to have made an active avoidance response to a conditioned stimulus (the buzzer). When treated with barbiturates above a certain dose, animals such as the rat are generally unable to make either the avoidance or the escape response and therefore they continue to receive the shock. The phenothiazines, on the other hand, have a more selective effect, interfering with avoidance behavior but not unconditioned escape responding. This test, with its separation of behaviors into conditioned and unconditioned components, subsequently has become the prototype procedure for the screening of potentially useful antipsychotic drugs.

The effect of the phenothiazines on avoidance behavior may possibly be due to a decrease in "vigilance" since something akin to this has been demonstrated in human studies involving continuous performance over long periods of time (e.g., pursuit-rotor test) wherein the individual must remain alert and vigilant to complete the task successfully. Although chlorpromazine significantly impairs such behavior, it does not appear to affect simple intellectual functioning such as that required on the digit-symbol substitution test. This experimental finding reflects the fact that in the treatment of psychotic behavior, chlorpromazine causes sedation but does not impair judgment. By contrast, secobarbital tends to interfere more with performance on tests measuring intellectual functioning than those measuring vigilance (Mirsky and Kornetsky, 1968).

Laboratory studies with chlorpromazine also reflect one of the other characteristic effects of this drug, namely, the "taming" of aggressive behavior. This is particularly dramatic in cases of "sham rage," which occur when experimental animals are lesioned in certain areas of the brain such as the diencephalon. The effect of these lesions is that the animal becomes violent and hyperaggressive, being provoked easily by the most innocuous stimuli. When treated with chlorpromazine, however, even in very low doses such as 0.1 mg/kg, animals once again become docile. This taming effect is also evident when violent patients are treated with this drug.

Chlorpromazine reduces motor activity in humans and animals in proportion to drug dosage. In fact, with rather high doses, chlorpromazine produces a cataleptic-like effect such that the various limbs of the body can be easily moved. In the laboratory, the effect of the phenothiazines in suppressing activity is especially observable in animals that have been made hyperactive with amphetamine. This suppressant effect is highly specific to the phenothiazines, suggesting that along with the active avoidance test situation, suppression of amphetamine-induced motor activity may be yet another useful screening device for the identification of antipsychotic agents (cf. Munkvad et al., 1968).

Related to this attenuating effect on spontaneous activity, however, is a characteristic extrapyramidal side effect which is often observable following chronic administration of the major tranquilizers. These extrapyramidal effects may include speech difficulties and actual muscle spasms; however, the overall advantages of treatment with these drugs far outweigh the undesirable side effects.

Judging from the fact that chlorpromazine does not affect intellectual functioning, it appears that the cortex is not one of its main sites of action. On the other hand, it has been shown that chlorpromazine does affect the activity of the reticular activating system, although this effect appears to be much different from that produced by the barbiturates. For example, whereas the latter group of drugs suppresses arousal stemming from both peripheral sensory stimulation and direct electrical stimulation, chlorpromazine exercises a more selective effect since only sensory input to the reticular system is suppressed (Killam, 1968). Whether this occurs as a result of some direct action on the reticular system itself or whether the effect is due to the actions of the drug on sensory relays has not been settled as yet.

The fact that the "sham rage" reaction is also suppressed indicates that the hypothalamus may be another main site of action for these drugs since "sham rage" arises primarily as a result of damage to this area of the brain. The probability of the hypothalamus being affected is supported further by the disruption of temperature regulation that also occurs following administration of these drugs. The result of this impairment is the development of poikilothermia such that the ability to control body temperature independent of the environment is impaired. This means that patients treated with chlorpromazine in climates with high temperatures may become hyperthermic as a result of their inability to lose body heat. By contrast, patients receiving the same medication in a cold climate may become hypothermic due to their impaired ability to preserve bodily heat.

The phenothiazines appear to be absorbed readily from gastrointestinal and parenteral sites of administration. Following absorption, they are distributed by the blood to the various tissues of the body, with the brain receiving less drug than the other organs of the body. The drug is subsequently metabolized through a number of different pathways and is eventually excreted via the kidney. The actual effect of these drugs on the nerve cell itself appears to involve several different mechanisms. One of these is an inhibition of oxidative phosphorylation and interference with utilization of ATP (see p. 8), possibly due to interference with the activity of mitochondria (Murray and Peterson, 1964). The phenothiazines are also known to exert a blockade of α-adrenergic receptors in the autonomic nervous system, and it has been suggested that they may selectively affect the adrenergic pathways of the ascending reticular system in the same way.

A second group of major tranquilizers are the rauwolfia alkaloids of which reserpine (Serpasil) is the prototype. Like the phenothiazines, reserpine exerts a calming effect on hitherto agitated psychotic behavior. The taming effect in animals is particularly striking. Overly aggressive monkeys, for example, become calm and quiescent after receiving this drug, but they can still be aroused by sensory stimuli and they will eat if they are hungry and provided with food. As with the phenothiazines, reserpine also blocks conditioned avoidance behavior but does not interfere with escape responding.

Although reserpine induces sleep, the kind of sleep is different from natural sleep in that it is characterized initially by a depression of both REM and nonREM activity (see p. 177). REM sleep begins to increase after the first few doses of reserpine, however, and this increase sometimes results in "nightmares."

The effects of reserpine on the CNS are rather complex and defy any simple explanation. At low doses, the activity of the reticular activating system is increased, but as the dosage is raised, reticular activity is inhibited. Activity in the cortex seems to be suppressed as well. The hypothalamus appears to be one of the primary sites of action since the "sham rage" response is suppressed readily by reserpine (cf. Weiskrantz and Wilson, 1955). Other changes that tend to occur are quite similar to those that follow stimulation of the posterior hypothalamus (i.e., sympathetic activity rather than parasympathetic), suggesting that this is the area of the hypothalamus most affected by the drug.

Reserpine's mechanism of action has been reviewed already (see p. 160) and therefore it is only outlined in this section. Basically, the rauwolfia drugs deplete norepinephrine, dopamine, and serotonin from their cellular storage sites in the brain and these changes have been regarded as the basis for their tranquilizing activity. However, it is not clear as yet whether it is the depletion of one of these amines or all three that is directly involved in the antipsychotic effects of these drugs.

The absorption and distribution of reserpine from oral and parenteral sites of administration occur fairly rapidly, although the onset of action, even with intravenous injection, is somewhat delayed, for example, 10 to 20 minutes. In addition, the effects of this drug persist long after it has been metabolized and eliminated from the body.

Although it was once used rather widely, reserpine is no longer administered to any great extent in the treatment of psychotic behavior due to its many adverse effects. For instance, in addition to its extrapyramidal activity, reserpine can also cause severe mental depression, headaches, dizziness, and nightmares.

A third class of major tranquilizers that has recently been introduced for the treatment of psychotic behavior is the butyrophenones, the prototype of which is haloperidol. According to Janssen and co-workers (e.g., Haase and Janssen, 1965) these are the most effective agents presently known for the treatment of schizophrenia characterized by hyperactivity and paranoid delusions. Much of the clinical literature now available tends to bear out this conclusion.

In animals, besides inhibiting conditioned avoidance behavior, haloperidol also suppresses the stereotypical increase in activity produced by amphetamine and the stereotypical gnawing behavior produced by apomorphine. On the basis of this latter effect, one of the main sites of action for these drugs appears to be the emetic trigger zone in the medulla. Among its other effects are a suppression of spontaneous motor activity at low doses and an induction of catalepsy at high doses (cf. Janssen, 1967). Haloperidol also appears to be more selective in its effects on the reticular system than the phenothiazines and rauwolfias since these latter drugs act on both the caudal and the rostral areas of this system, whereas haloperidol affects only the caudal portion.

Haloperidol is absorbed readily from both gastrointestinal and parenteral sites of injection. It is metabolized in the liver and excreted via the kidneys. Its mechanism of action at the cellular level has been attributed to a blockade of dopamine receptors (van Rossum, 1967). This hypothesis is based in part upon the fact that haloperidol antagonizes the hyperactivity effects of amphetamine which are mediated through dopaminergic pathways, and in part on the observation of a direct antagonism of the fall in blood pressure produced by dopamine following blockade of sympathetic adrenergic receptors in the cat (van Rossum, 1967). Another line of evidence implicating haloperidol as a dopamine receptor blocking agent is the fact that it is able to antagonize the hypothermic effects of apomorphine, a compound with relatively specific dopamine receptor stimulant properties (cf. Barnett et al., 1972). For example, Fig. 5.8 shows that haloperidol shifts the dose-response curve for apomorphine to the right, thus demonstrating haloperidol's competitive antagonism properties. In light of such evidence, it has been suggested that the etiology of schizophrenia may in some way be related to an excess of dopamine in the CNS (Stein and Wise, 1971).

Whatever the mechanism of action of these drugs, however, it is readily apparent that the major tranquilizers have proved themselves one of the most useful aids presently available for the treatment of aberrant behavior. More often than not, psychotic behavior is arrested and individuals that hitherto were apathetic and unresponsive to traditional forms of psychotherapy have become more amenable to such treatment following administration of these drugs. As a result, they can often leave the confines of the hospital for the community clinic where they can participate in rehabilitation programs on an out-patient basis. In such cases, the prognosis for

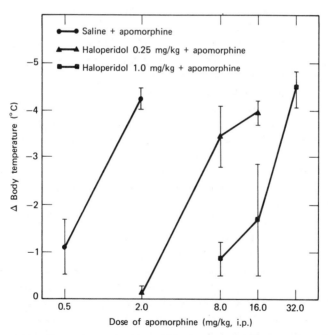

Fig. 5.8 Antagonism of apomorphine-induced hypothermia by haloperidol. Each point represents the mean ± S.E. of five mice. The results were obtained 30 minutes after apomorphine and 60 minutes after haloperidol (from Barnett et al., 1972).

their eventual recovery is far greater than would be the case were they to remain hospitalized.

Minor Tranquilizers

The minor tranquilizers are used to treat behavioral disorders called neuroses which often emerge as a consequence of unresolved conflicts. Unlike the psychotic, the neurotic has not lost contact with reality. His main problem is uncontrollable anxiety and tension. The neurotic is someone who is constantly apprehensive, often without knowing exactly what it is he is actually apprehensive about.

One of the first drugs to be used widely for the treatment of neurotic behavior was meprobamate (Miltown). Although it was administered initially for its muscle relaxant properties, it was observed that this drug also alleviated feelings of anxiety and tension. However, meprobamate was not found tranquilizing enough to be useful in the treatment of psychotic disorders. Unlike the phenothiazines, or the other antipsychotic drugs, it also does not selectively suppress conditioned avoidance behavior nor does it produce any of the extrapyramidal effects characteristic of the major tranquilizers. In addition, meprobamate also differs from the sedative-hypnotic group of drugs in several ways. For example, in comparing meprobamate and the barbiturates, Berger (1963) reported that whereas the barbiturates slowed EEG activity to less than 6 cps, meprobamate hardly ever reduced EEG frequencies to such low levels, even following administration of near toxic dosages. Meprobamate, in fact, appears to have little direct effect on any part of the CNS. Instead, its therapeutic value appears to lie directly in its muscle-relaxant properties. This phenomenon of ameliorating neurotic problems via muscle relaxation is in keeping with the work of Jacobson (1938), the leading proponent of the method of "progressive relaxation." According to his views, all emotional problems involve the contraction of muscles. Because this contraction causes the stimulation of proprioceptors throughout the body (see p. 40), it results in a tremendous increase in the neural activity of the brain. By a person's learning to relax, Jacobson argues, the amount of nervous input can be attenuated and as a result nervous tension will be reduced. Apparently a drug such as meprobamate which is able to relax skeletal muscles is likewise able to decrease the amount of proprioceptive stimulation to the brain; if Jacobson is correct, this would appear to be the basis for its therapeutic value.

Meprobamate itself is absorbed readily from both gastrointestinal and parenteral administration sites. No localization of the drug occurs in any particular area of the CNS. About 10% remains unchanged and is excreted via the kidneys; the rest of the drug is metabolized by the liver.

Like the barbiturates, chronic use of meprobamate will result in tolerance due to induced hepatic enzyme activity (Phillips et al., 1962). Physical dependence is also known to occur following chronic usage of high doses (more than 1.5 g/day). Among the symptoms that develop in man during abstinence are hallucinations, anxiety, convulsions, coma, and possibly death. In mice, abstinence symptoms marked by heightened excitability have been observed as early as 4 hours after withdrawal. By comparison, the abstinence syndrome which follows withdrawal from chronic alcohol or phenobarbital usage does not occur until about 24 hours after the last administration of these drugs (Domino, 1971).

The benzodiazepines chiefly represented by chlordiazepoxide (Librium), diazepam (Valium), and oxazepam (Serax) are a second group of antianxiety drugs which appear to owe much of their efficacy to their skeletal muscle-relaxant properties. Apparently by depressing spinal reflex activity, neural activity in the brain stem reticular activating system is reduced (Przbyla and Wang, 1968) and activity in the cortex is also attenuated.

Like meprobamate and the barbiturates, these drugs do not selectively impair conditioned avoidance behavior indicating that they lack efficacy as antipsychotic agents. Another characteristic they share with meprobamate and the barbiturates is the taming action they exert on aggression in both monkeys and mice that have been stimulated to fight by applying shock to their feet. However, unlike the barbiturates and meprobamate, they do so at doses that do not produce any effects on spontaneous activity (Randall et al., 1961).

Although the benzodiazepines are absorbed from both gastrointestinal and parenteral sites, peak plasma levels are not attained until about 8 hours after injection. The duration of action, however, is rather prolonged, that of chlordiazepoxide being longer than that of diazepam, which in turn is longer than that of oxazepam. The latter is, in fact, a metabolite of diazepam. In general, the blood levels of these drugs tend to remain rather high for several days after treatment, the half-life in the blood being about 24 hours. Inactivation occurs via several different metabolic routes and elimination occurs through the kidneys.

At low doses, there is little possibility for the development of tolerance or physical dependence with these drugs. However, should very high doses be taken over a prolonged period of time, both tolerance and physical dependence will occur (Hollister et al., 1961). The benzodiazepines are in fact subject to chronic usage because they tend to engender a heightened sense of well-being in which the user almost appears to be inebriated. Another side effect which sometimes accompanies use of these drugs is a sudden increase in appetite such that the individual begins to eat voraciously (Jarvik, 1970).

ANTIDEPRESSANTS

One of the more commonly encountered emotional disorders for which drugs are prescribed often is depression. This is a condition in which there is an overwhelming sense of sadness and melancholy. The depressed individual appears to have lost interest in everything. He has no desire for food and suffers an attendant weight loss. There is also a loss of sexual interests and concern with work. The depressed individual is unable to make decisions or concentrate on any problems except those concerning his own morbidity.

Until the 1950s, the main treatment for this disorder was electroconvulsive shock therapy. This produced dramatic improvements, but because of the frightening convulsions and the amnesia that often occurs following such treatment, other means of remedy have largely replaced this kind of treatment. The two main chemical forms of therapy that have been adopted are the monoamine oxidase inhibitors and the tricyclic antidepressants.

The mechanism of action of the MAO inhibitors has been reviewed already (see p. 34) and therefore only a brief summary is repeated here. Basically, the main action of these compounds is to reduce the activity of monoamine oxidase, the enzyme responsible for the metabolic degradation of norepinephrine, dopamine, and serotonin. Following inhibition of MAO, the concentration of these amines in the brain is elevated markedly. Thus, whereas reserpine causes sedation by means of reducing amine levels in the brain, the MAO inhibitors cause stimulation as a result of increasing their concentration. This observation has given rise to the so-called "catecholamine hypothesis," which contends that depression itself is a function of the concentration of these amines, particularly norepinephrine, in the CNS.

Because the concept of depression is rather subjective, it has been rather difficult to devise experimental techniques to test this hypothesis in animals. One experimental procedure that appears to have some potential in this regard, however, involves the self-stimulation technique introduced by Olds and Milner (1954). In using this method, electrodes are implanted in certain areas of the brain such as the limbic system or the hypothalamus. By pressing a lever, an animal is then able to direct electrical current to these areas. The effect of such a consequence is that the animal will press the lever for more than 1000 times per hour in order to stimulate his brain in this manner. This observation has led to the hypothesis that these areas of the CNS in which electrical stimulation of this sort is able to reinforce such behavior constitute the neural pathways for "pleasure" in the brain. This hypothesis has been developed further by Stein (1962), who suggests that in depression, these "pleasure" areas have become hypoactive due to a diminution of the neurotransmitter's mediating activity in the pleasure pathways. In this regard, pharmacological investigations involving the administration of catecholamine-affecting drugs have indicated that the neurotransmitter in these pathways is adrenergic in nature, and therefore the basis for depression may involve a decrease in the concentration of adrenergic transmitters in these "pleasure zones." This hypothesis has been supported further by experiments that demonstrate that drugs which are MAO inhibitors are able to increase the rate of responding for self-stimulation at doses that do not affect spontaneous motor activity (Poschel and Ninteman, 1963, 1964).

Among the best known of the MAO inhibitors are tranylcypromine (Parnate), pargyline (Eutonyl), isocarboxazid (Marplan), nialamide (Niamid), and phenelzine sulfate (Nardil). These drugs are absorbed rapidly from both gastrointestinal and parenteral sites, but they do not produce their maximal effects until about 24 hours or more after their administration. Although they are eliminated rapidly from the body, their effects are rather long-lasting owing to the fact that they irreversibly inactivate monoamine oxidase.

The MAO inhibitors are no longer widely used in clinical practice, however, because they can be highly toxic. Although damage to the liver was often reported with some of the early MAO inhibitors, the risk of liver damage has now been reduced markedly, but the danger has not been completely overcome. In addition, because of their stimulant properties, administration of these drugs may also be followed by irritability, restlessness, confusion, and insomnia. It is for this reason that usage of these drugs has been replaced by the group of drugs known as the tricyclic antidepressants.

The best known of this latter class of compounds are imipramine (Toframil), desipramine (Norpramin), and amitriptyline (Elavil). The mechanism of action of these drugs appears to involve a reduction in the reuptake of norepinephrine by adrenergic neurons after it has been released from its synaptic terminals. This hypothesis is based on the observation that imipramine lowers the concentration of norepinephrine in tissues but increases its concentration in the blood (Axelrod et al., 1961). Because of this interference with the uptake mechanism, more transmitter is available to adrenergic receptors, and apparently this is the basis for the antidepressant effect of these drugs. In this regard, one of the characteristic effects of this group of drugs is their ability to antagonize and to reverse the sedative and hypothermic effects of monoamine releasing drugs such as reserpine.

The tricyclics are absorbed quickly from their sites of administration and they are distributed rapidly to the brain as indicated by the speed with which their effects can be observed. These drugs are also metabolized and eliminated rather quickly from the body. Among the adverse side effects that sometimes accompany their usage, however, are hallucinations, delusions, and hyperexcitability. It is because of this latter effect that these drugs are sometimes classified as CNS stimulants.

ANALGESICS

Drugs that fall into this category cause the relief of pain without producing general anesthesia. With drugs such as morphine, there is no actual diminution of sensation; what is affected is the "psychological" response to pain. The fact that psychological factors play an important role in the reaction to pain is readily apparent from clinical records showing that during wartime 25% of the hospitalized battle-wounded patients requested morphine for their injuries, compared with an 80% rate for civilian hospitalized patients. Seemingly, the explanation for this phenomenon lies in the way each individual perceived his pain. For the soldier, his wound was a welcome ticket home; for the civilian patient, pain was an unpleasantry that he chose not to tolerate. Thus pain has both sensory and perceptual sides. The fact that pain can be produced by the excitation of specific fibers which do not also signal other sensations indicates that there is indeed a dsitinct sensory component to pain. The fact that the perception of such stimuli can be modified if other sensory stimuli are simultaneously presented along with a pain stimulus supports somewhat the argument that pain has a perceptual side as well.

The local anesthetics discussed above are examples of drugs which act on the stimulus aspect of pain. Local anesthetics are able to perform this function because they are capable of blocking nerve conduction. The analgesics, on the other hand, are compounds which affect the perceptual aspect of pain. The latter group of drugs is usually subdivided into the narcotic analgesics depress activtiy in the CNS in addition to their analgesic activity, whereas the nonnarcotic analgesics do not. Because the nonnarcotic analgesics for example, aspirin, phenacetin, and antipyrine, do not have major behavioral effects, they are not included in further discussion of the analgesic drugs.

The main narcotic analgesics are morphine and codeine. Both are alkaloid derivatives of opium. Heroin (diacetylmorphine) is not found in opium but is produced by causing a slight change in the chemical structure of morphine. This enables it to pass through the blood-brain barrier much faster and therefore in greater concentrations per unit time than is the case with equivalent doses of morphine. Once in the brain, however, heroin is metabolized back into morphine. In addition to the naturally occurring narcotic analgesics, a number of synthetic narcotic analgesics also have been developed, the best known of which is meperidine (Demerol).

The analgesic activity of the opium derivatives is due to their actions on both the sensory and perceptual components of pain. On the stimulus side, the threshold for excitation of pain fibers is increased slightly, but not markedly. More important is their effect on the perception of pain stimuli. After receiving morphine, subjects are still able to feel pain but they report being indifferent to it. In this respect, the narcotic analgesics are much more specific in their mechanism of action than are the general anesthetics. The exact nature by which this effect is accomplished, however, is still problematical. At present, the most likely explanation is that its action on pain perception is due mainly to a calming, fear-reducing effect. Animal experiments, however, indicate that "emotionality" in general appears to be reduced. For example, when morphine is given to animals, the rates of lever pressing for electrical stimulation directed either to the "pleasure" or "pain" centers of the brain are both decreased (Olds and Travis, 1960; Vernier et al., 1961). This suggests that in some way, morphine may act indiscriminately on the neural pathways underlying "emotionality."

In addition to its pain-alleviating properties, morphine is also known to produce a marked sense of euphoria and well-being in certain individuals. It is because of these pleasurable sensations that morphine and its analogues are subject to abuse. However, it should be pointed out that although addicts often describe the effects of intravenous injections of these drugs in terms of an orgasm, controlled clinical studies indicate that this is not a general reaction since many people often experience a sense of unpleasantness and nausea following the same kind of treatment. This latter experience of dysphoria has been attributed by some to the clinical setting in which the experiments are conducted, but this explanation does not appear to be valid since information from street addicts tends to corroborate the finding that morphine-like drugs often produce feelings that are opposite to those for which their usage was intended (cf. Isbell and White, 1953).

The opioid drugs are absorbed readily from parenteral sites but absorption from the gastrointestinal tract is not as good. Because its effects are attenuated following administration by the oral route, morphine is commonly administered intramuscularly or intravenously ("mainlining"). Although the main site of action is in the CNS, only small amounts of morphine actually pass the blood-brain barrier. Nevertheless, it appears that only a minute amount of this drug must be present in the brain for its effects to be experienced. Most of the drug is metabolized in the liver and is excreted via the kidney. At present there is no generally accepted hypothesis concerning the cellular site of action of these drugs. It is generally agreed, however, that specific neuronal receptors respond to the presence of these drugs. The basis for this assumption is the fact that the effects of the opioids can be blocked by specific antagonists such as naloxone. Although these postulated receptors are different from those at which neurotransmitters act, it does appear that the opioids in some way also affect synaptic transmission. The transmitter substance that seems to be mainly affected in producing morphine's analgesic effects is serotonin, whereas norepinephrine seems to be the transmitter involved in its euphoria-producing properties.

The motivation for self-administration of the narcotic analgesics is reputed to be the sense of euphoria that they induce. Associated with this feeling, however, is an indifference to social concerns and a reduction in the frequency of occurrence of behaviors involving hunger, sex, work, etc. Constipation, pupillary constriction, nausea, vomiting, and changes in body temperatures are some of the physiological concomitants associated with the use of these drugs.

With the exception of constipation and pupillary constriction, marked tolerance develops to most of these effects so that the user must continue to increase the dosage of these drugs in order to achieve the same pleasurable effects he initially sought in their usage. However, the primary motivation for continued administration of these drugs by chronic users is often that of preventing the aversiveness associated with withdrawal. It is important to note, however, that an individual must usually administer these drugs to himself several times a day for several days for dependence to occur. Neither tolerance nor physical dependence usually develops after a single injection in man.

Although increased metabolism and cellular adaptation have both been suggested as explanations for the development of tolerance to these drugs, each suggestion has been contradicted by experimental findings (see Murphree, 1971). Apparently, some as yet unknown mechanism is responsible for these effects. Physical dependence on the opioids becomes evident about 12 hours after the last administration of these drugs, with peak activity becoming manifest about 48 to 72 hours after withdrawal. These effects increase progressively in intensity and adversity, beginning with restlessness, irritability, tremors, lacrimation, nausea, vomiting, diarrhea, chills alternating with execess sweating, abdominal cramps, and spasms and kicking movements. These symptoms may last as long as 10 days from the beginning of abstinence.

As mentioned above, there are a number of compounds that are able to antagonize many of the effects of the narcotic analgesics. Some of these also possess analgesic activity themselves, suggesting that both the narcotic analgesics and the narcotic antagonists act upon the same receptor sites and that, although the latter have greater affinity for these receptors, the former have greater intrinsic activity (see p. 107).

The main narcotic antagonists presently in use are methadone, nalorphine, pentazocine, cyclazocine, and naloxone. All these compounds have analgesic activity of their own, however, except for naloxone, which has minimal analgesic activity and therefore comes closest to being a "pure" antagonist. Some of the major uses of these narcotic antagonists are directed at blocking the effects of morphine and heroin. For example, the narcotic antagonists are often administered to reverse the effects of an

states. The possible involvement of certain neurotransmitters in the etiology of schizophrenia has already been noted in connection with the "catecholamine hypothesis" of affective disorders (see p. 190). In this regard, it has been suggested that the mechanism of action of the psychotomimetics may in some way involve their tendency either to mimic the effects of certain amines or else interfere with their normal metabolic inactivation. For example, there are certain marked similarities in structure between mescaline and epinephrine and between LSD and serotonin. It is usually conceded, however, that the actual experience which results from the use of these drugs depends upon many factors such as the expectations of the individual, his familiarity with the drug, his feelings at the time of drug usage, and the setting in which the drug is taken. It is because these feelings are so important, in that they tend to be enhanced by these compounds, that the term "psychedelic" or "mind expanding" is often used to describe them. Indeed, the main characteristic of these drugs is said to be their capacity to enable the user to detect and to respond to sources of stimulus input that might otherwise be too subtle to discriminate. As a consequence of this enhancement, new perceptions are experienced along with a greater incidence of illusions and, occasionally, hallucinations. It is with respect to this latter experience, in fact, that these drugs are sometimes referred to as hallucinogens in the sense that the user reports being able to see or hear stimuli along unique dimensions. For example, one kind of perceptual anomaly that is often reported is synesthesia, that is, the ability to hear colors and see sounds. Hallucinogen is an inappropriate term, however, since these drugs seldom produce true hallucinations in the sense of the user reporting the perception of stimuli that are not actually physically present.

MESCALINE

This is the active component of the peyote cactus (*Lophophora williamsii*). The name mescaline is derived from the Mescalero Apache Indians who used it extensively in their religious ceremonies. The effects produced by this compound are usually twofold. At first a rather unpleasant sensation— for example, anxiety, nausea, and tremors—is experienced for about 1 to 2 hours after ingestion (the usual oral dose is about 5 mg/kg). This is then followed by a dream-like sensation characterized primarily by vivid visual hallucinations lasting several hours.

LSD

d-lysergic acid diethylamide (LSD) is produced by combining diethylamide with lysergic acid, a substance extracted from the fungus *Claviceps pur-*

purea. Although LSD was synthesized in the late 1930s, it was not until 1943 that its peculiar behavioral properties were discovered. The occasion for this discovery was the accidental ingestion of a minute quantity of this compound by A. Hofmann, a research chemist working at the Sandoz laboratories in Basel, Switzerland. Among the sensations experienced by Hofmann were dizziness, perceptual distortions, and visual hallucinations. Because this discovery was made during wartime, however, these results were not made known until several years later (Stoll, 1947). Since then, more than a thousand research papers dealing with the properties of this compound have appeared in the scientific literature.

LSD is a very potent compound. For example, 50 μg/kg of body weight is enough to produce its characteristic effects in humans. Absorption is fairly rapid from both gastrointestinal and parenteral sites of administration. Distribution is also fairly rapid although it appears that very little of the drug actually enters the brain (Axelrod et al., 1957). The duration of action lasts about 6 to 8 hours and elimination occurs via the kidney.

Once the drug enters the brain, the reticular activating system appears to be a main site of action. The effect is one of sensitization (cf. Bradley and Elkes, 1953), in contrast to drugs such as chlorpromazine, which reduces the responsiveness of this system to sensory stimulation. Because LSD has been shown to be a potent antagonist of serotonin (Gaddum and Hameed, 1954), it has been suggested that this antagonism may be the basis for its behavioral effects. However, neither 2-bromo-LSD nor methysergide, which are both potent inhibitors of serotonin, produce any comparable effects on behavior. At present, LSD's mechanism of action is therefore still problematical. Before passing on to the next drug, it should also be noted that tolerance to the behavioral effects of LSD develops rather rapidly if the doses are taken repeatedly within a short time of one another.

PSILOCYBIN

This is the active ingredient in the Psilocybe mushroom. As with mescaline, it was used for many centuries by various Indian tribes as part of their religious ceremonies. Psilocybin is absorbed readily from both gastrointestinal and parenteral sites and in general it produces an initially unpleasant effect analogous to that produced by mescaline. This is then followed by the sensation of perceptual distortions. For the most part, however, psilocybin has not been studied to the same extent as have the preceding drugs, and so less is known concerning its effects at the behavioral level. It is interesting to note, however, that cross-tolerance between psilocybin and LSD has been observed (Isbell et al., 1961), suggesting that these two drugs share some basic mechanism of action in common.

MARIHUANA

This refers to the hemp plant, *Cannabis sativa.* The active material in marihuana has now been isolated and identified as delta-9-tetrahydrocannabinol (Δ^9-THC). As with many of the other psychotomimetic drugs, marihuana had been used for many centuries before it came to the attention of the scientific community.

Marihuana is usually smoked in the form of a cigarette. In this way, its active principle is taken directly into the lungs and from there it quickly enters the bloodstream, the effects becoming recognizable within 5 minutes of administration. In general, a feeling of euphoria and well-being is produced. Although it has been claimed that sensory acuity is improved, all experimental attempts thus far have failed to support this assertion. The response to the drug is in fact quite variable. Among those behavioral effects which do appear valid and which have been documented are distortions of time perception, memory, and feelings of insatiable hunger (cf. Abel, 1971). This latter effect appears to be particularly human since experiments with animals usually have produced diametrically opposite results.

At present, the mechanism of action for Δ^9-THC is unknown. Even hazarding a guess along these lines is particularly difficult since it does not have a chemical structure which resembles any of the other psychotomimetics or any known neurochemical, nor have its effects been reversed by any known pharmacological antagonist.

Bibliography

Abel, E. L. Habituation As A Factor In Early Handling. *Journal of Comparative and Physiological Psychology*, 1971, **74**, 219–221. (*a*).

Abel, E. L. Effects of Marihuana on the Solution of Anagrams, Memory, and Appetite. *Nature*, 1971, **231**, 260–261. (*b*)

Abel, E. L. Marihuana and Memory: Acquisition or Retrieval? *Science*, 1971, **73**, 1038–1040. (*c*)

Abel, E. L. *Ancient Views on the Origins of Life*. Fairleigh Dickinson University Press, Madison, N.J., 1973.

Abel, E. L., McMillan, D. E., and Harris, L. S. Tolerance to the Hypothermic Effects of Δ^9-Tetrahydrocannabinol as a Function of Age in the Chicken. *British Journal of Pharmacology*, 1973, **47**, 452–456.

Abel, E. L., McMillan, D. E., and Harris, L. S. Δ^9-Tetrahydrocannabinol: Effects of Route of Administration on Onset and Duration of Activity and Tolerance Development. *Psychopharmacologia*, 1974, **35**, 29–38.

Ahlquist, R. P. A Study of the Adrenotropic Receptors. *American Journal of Physiology*, 1948, **153**, 586–600.

Ahlquist, R. P. Agents Which Block Adrenergic β-Receptors. *Annual Review of Pharmacology*, 1968, **8**, 259–272.

Anderson, K. W. The Oral Absorption of Quinalbarbitone and Its Sodium Salt. *Archives Internationales de Pharmacodynamie et de Thérapie*, 1964, **147**, 171–177.

Anderson, P., Eccles, J. C., and Loyning, Y. Pathway of Postsynaptic Inhibition in the Hippocampus. *Journal of Physiology*, 1964, **172**, 608–619. (*a*)

Anderson, P., Eccles, J. C., and Sears, T. A. The Ventro-Basal Complex Of The Thalamus: Types of Cells, Their Responses And Their Functional Organization. *Journal of Physiology*, 1964, **174**, 370–399. (*b*)

Andrews, H. L. Changes in the Electroencephalogram During a Cycle of Morphine Addiction. *Psychosomatic Medicine*, 1943, **5**, 143–147.

Anton, A. H. The Relations Between the Binding of Sulfonamides to Albumin and Their Antibacterial Efficacy. *Journal of Pharmacology and Experimental Therapeutics*, 1960, **129**, 282–290.

Arias, I. M., Gartner, L., Furman, M., and Wolfson, S. Effects of Several Drugs and Chemicals on Hepatic Glucuronide Formation in Newborn Rats. *Proceedings of the Society for Experimental Biology and Medicine*, 1963, **112**, 1037–1040.

Ariens, E. J. Affinity and Intrinsic Activity in the Theory of Competitive Inhibition. *Archives Internationales de Pharmacodynamie et de Thérapie*, 1954, **99**, 32–50.

Ariens, E. J. Receptor Theory and Structure-Action Relationships. *Advances in Drug Research*, 1966, **3**, 235–285.

Aschoff, J. Circadian Rhythm of Activity and of Body Temperature. In *Physiological And Behavioral Temperature Regulation*. J. D. Hardy, A. P. Gagge, and J. A. J. Stolwijk (Eds.). Charles C Thomas, Springfield, Ill., 1970.

Astatoor, A. M., Galman, B. R., Johnson, J. R., and Milne, J. D. The Excretion of Dexamphetamine and its Derivatives. *British Journal of Pharmacology*, 1965, **24**, 293–300.

Aston, R. Acute Tolerance Indices For Pentobarbital In Male and Female Rats. *Journal of Pharmacology and Experimental Therapeutics*, 1966, **152**, 350–353.

Axelrod, J., Brady, R. O., Witkop, B., and Evarts, E. V. The Distribution and Metabolism of Lysergic Acid Diethylamide. *Annals of the New York Academy of Sciences*, 1957, **66**, 435–444.

Axelrod, J., Reichenthal, J., and Brodie, B. B. Mechanism of the Potentiating Action of β-Diethylaminoethyl Diphenylpropylacetate. *Journal of Pharmacology and Experimental Therapeutics*, 1954, **112**, 49–54.

Axelrod, J., Whitby, L. G., and Hertling, G. Effect of Psychotropic Drugs on the Uptake of H^3-Norepinephrine by Tissues. *Science*. 1961, **133**, 383–384.

Bagdon, W. J., and Mann, D. E. Chlorpromazine Hyperthermia in Young Albino Mice. *Journal of Pharmaceutical Sciences*, 1962, **51**, 753–755.

Bainbridge, J. G. The Inhibitory Effect of Amphetamine on Exploration in Mice. *Psychopharmacologia*, 1970, **18**, 314–319.

Bakay, L. Studies On The Blood-Brain Barrier With Radioactive Phosphorus. *Archives of Neurology and Psychiatry*, 1951, **66**, 419–426.

Bakay, L. Dynamic Aspects Of The Blood-Brain Barrier. In *Metabolism Of The Nervous System*, D. Richter (Ed.). Permagon Press, New York, 1957.

Ballard, B. E. Biopharmaceutical Considerations in Subcutaneous and Intramuscular Drug Administration. *Journal of Pharmaceutical Sciences*, 1968, **57**, 357–378.

Ban, T. A. *Psychopharmacology*, Williams and Wilkins, Baltimore, 1969.

Barger, G., and Dale, H. H. Chemical Structure and Sympathomimetic Action of Amines. *Journal of Physiology*, 1910, **41**, 19–59.

Barnes, J. M., and Trueto, J. Absorption of Bacteria, Toxins and Snake Venoms from the Tissues. *Lancet*, **1941**(1), 623–626.

Barnett, A., Goldstein, J., and Taber, R. I. Apomorphine-Induced Hypothermia in Mice; A Possible Dopaminergic Effect. *Archives Internationales de Pharmacodynamie et de Thérapie*, 1972, **198**, 242–247.

Bastian, J. W. Classification of CNS Drugs by a Mouse Screening Battery. *Archives Internationales de Pharmacodynamie et de Thérapie*, 1961, **133**, 347–364.

Battey, L. L., Heyman, A., and Patterson, J. L. Effect of Ethyl Alcohol on Cerebral Blood Flow and Metabolism. *Journal of the American Medical Association*, 1953, **152**, 6–10.

Beckett, A. H., Rowland, M., and Turner, P. Influence of Urinary pH on Excretion of Amphetamine. *Lancet*, **1965**(1), 303.

Belleau, B. Conformational Perturbation in Relation to the Regulation of Enzyme and Receptor Behavior. *Advances in Drug Research*, 1965, **2**, 89–126.

Berger, F. M. The Similarities and Differences between Meprobamate and Barbiturates. *Clinical Pharmacology and Therapeutics*, 1963, **4**, 209–231.

Bertler, A., and Rosengren, E. Occurrence and Distribution of Catecholamines in Brain. *Acta Physiologica Scandinavica*, 1959, **47**, 350–361.

Bhagat, B. D., *Recent Advances in Adrenergic Mechanisms*. Charles C Thomas, Springfield, Ill., 1971.

Bhargava, K. P., Dhawan, K. N., and Saxena, R. C. Enhancement of Noradrenaline Pressor Responses on Testosterone-Treated Cats. *British Journal of Pharmacology*, 1967, **31**, 26–31.

Black, R. W., Fowler, R. L., and Kimbrell, G. Adaptation and Habituation of Heart Rate to Handling in the Rat. *Journal of Comparative and Physiological Psychology*, 1964, **57**, 422–425.

Bloom, F. E., Oliver, A. P., and Salmoiraghi, G. C. The Responsiveness of Individual Hypothalamic Neurons to Microelectrophoretically Administered Endogenous Amines. *International Journal of Neuropharmacology*, 1963, **2**, 181–193.

Bogdanski, D. F., Weissbach, H., and Udenfriend, S. The Distribution of Serotonin, 5-Hydroxytryptophan Decarboxylase and Monoamine Oxidase in Brain. *Journal of Neurochemistry*, 1957, **1**, 272–278.

Bolles, R. C. Species-specific Defense Reactions and Avoidance Learning. *Psychological Review*, 1970, **77**, 32–48.

Booth, D. A., and Quartermain, D. Taste Sensitivity of Eating Elicited by Chemical Stimulation of the Rat Hypothalamus. *Psychonomic Science*, 1965, **3**, 525–526.

Borga, O., Azarnoff, D. L., and Sjoquist, F. Species Differences in the Plasma Protein Binding of Desipramine. *Journal of Pharmacy and Pharmacology*, 1968, **20**, 571–572.

Bradley, P. B. Synaptic Transmission in the Central Nervous System and Its Relevance for Drug Action. *International Review of Neurobiology*, 1968, **11**, 1–56.

Bradley, P. B., and Key, B. J. The Effect of Drugs on Arousal Responses Produced by Electrical Stimulation of the Reticular Formation of the Brain. *Electroencephalography and Clinical Neurophysiology*, 1958, **10**, 97–110.

Bradley, P. B., and Key, B. J. A Comparative Study of the Effects of Drugs on the Arousal System of the Brain. *British Journal of Pharmacology*, 1959, **14**, 340–349.

Bradley, P. B., Dhawan, B. N., and Wolstencroft, J. H. Pharmacological Properties of Cholinoceptive Neurones in the Medulla and Pons of the Cat. *Journal of Physiology*, 1966, **183**, 658–674.

Brochet, J. The Living Cell. *Scientific American*, 1961, **205**, 51–62.

Brodie, B. B. Physico-chemical Factors in Drug Absorption. In *Absorption and Distribution of Drugs*. T. B. Binns (Ed.). Williams and Wilkins, Baltimore, 1964, pp. 16–48. (*a*)

Brodie, B. B. Distribution and Fate of Drugs: Therapeutic Implications. In *Absorption and Distribution of Drugs*. T. B. Binns (Ed.). Williams and Wilkins, Baltimore, 1964, pp. 199–251. (*b*)

Brodie, B. B., and Hogben, C. A. M. Some Physiochemical Factors in Drug Action. *Journal of Pharmacy and Pharmacology*, 1957, **9**, 345–380.

Brodie, B. B., and Reid, W. D. The Value of Determining the Plasma Concentration of Drugs in Animals and Man. In *Fundamentals of Drug Metabolism and Drug Disposition*. B. N. LaDu, H. G. Mandel, and E. L. Way (Eds.). Williams and Wilkins, Baltimore, 1971.

Brodie, B. B., Spector, S., and Shore, P. A. Interaction of Drugs with Norepinephrine in the Brain. *Pharmacological Review,* 1959, **11**, 548–564.

Bünning, E. *The Physiological Clock*, Springer-Verlag, Berlin, 1964.

Burn, J. H., and Rand, M. J. A New Interpretation of the Adrenergic Nerve Fibre. *Advances in Pharmacology*, 1962, **1**, 1–30.

Burns, J. J. Variation of Drug Metabolism in Animals and the Prediction of Drug Action in Man. *Annals of the New York Academy of Sciences*, 1958, **151**, 959–967.

Burns, J. J., Berger, B. L., Lief, P. A., et al. The Physiological Disposition and Fate of Meperidine (Demerol) in Man and a Method for its Estimation in Plasma. *Journal of Pharmacology and Experimental Therapeutics*, 1955, **114**, 289–298.

Calesnick, B. Intimate Study of Drug Action. IV. In *Drill's Pharmacology in Medicine*. J. R. Dipalma (Ed.). McGraw-Hill, New York, 1965.

Calesnick, B. Practical Problems in Drug Dosage. *Seminars in Drug Treatment*, 1971, **1**, 63–91.

Canon, W. B. *The Wisdom of the Body*, W. W. Norton, New York, 1966.

Chance, M. R. A. Factors Influencing the Toxicity of Sympathomimetic Amines to Solitary Mice. *Journal of Pharmacology and Experimental Therapeutics*, 1947, **89**, 289–296.

Ciaccio, E. I. Intimate Study of Drug Action. II: Fate of Drugs in the Body. In *Drill's Pharmacology in Medicine*. J. R. Dipalma (Ed.). McGraw-Hill, New York, 1971.

Cicero, T. J., and Myers, R. D. Preference-Aversion Functions for Alcohol After Cholinergic Stimulation of the Brain and Fluid Deprivation. *Physiology and Behavior*, 1969, **4**, 559–562.

Clark, A. J. Methods of General Pharmacology. *Handbuch der experimentellen Pharmakologie*, 1947, **4**, 61–79.

Cochin, J. Some Aspects of Tolerance to the Narcotic Analgesics. In *Drug Addiction: Experimental Pharmacology*. J. M. Singh, L. Miller, and H. Lai (Eds.). Future Publishing Co., Mt. Kisco, N.Y., 1972, Vol. I, pp. 365–375.

Cochin, J., and Kornetsky, C. Development and Loss of Tolerance to Morphine in the Rat After Single and Multiple Injections. *Journal of Pharmacology and Experimental Therapeutics*, 1964, **145**, 1–10.

Cole, H. F., and Wolf, H. The Effects of Some Psychotropic Drugs on Conditioned Avoidance and Aggressive Behaviors. *Psychopharmacologia*, 1966, **8**, 389–396.

Cole, H. F., and Wolf, H. A Pharmacological Evaluation of a Genetically Predisposed Conditioned Avoidance Response. *Proceedings of the Society for Experimental Biology and Medicine*, 1969, **132**, 1067–1071.

Collier, H. O. J. Tolerance, Physical Dependence and Receptors. *Advances in Drug Research*, 1966, **3**, 171–188.

Cook, L., and Weidly, E. W. Behavioral Effects of Some Psychopharmacological Agents. *Annals of the New York Academy of Sciences*, 1957, **66**, 740–752.

Coons, E. E., and Quartermain, D. Motivational Depression Associated with Norepi-nephrine-induced Eating from the Hypothalamus; Resemblance to the Ventromedial Hyperphagic Syndrome. *Physiology and Behavior*, 1970, **5**, 687–692.

Cooper, J. R., Bloom, F. E., and Roth, R. H. *The Biochemical Basis of Neuropharmacology.* Oxford University Press, New York, 1970.

Crout, J. R. Effect of Inhibiting both Catechol-*o*-methyl Transferase and Monoamine Oxidase on Cardiovascular Responses to Norepinephrine. *Proceedings of the Society for Experimental Biology and Medicine*, 1961, **108**, 482–484.

Curtis, D. R. The Effect of Drugs adn Amino Acids upon Neutrons. In *Regional Neuro-chemistry*. S. S. Kety and J. Elkes (Eds.). Permagon Press, New York, 1961, pp. 403–422.

Dale, H. H. The Action of Certain Esters and Ethers of Choline, and their Relation to Muscarine. *Journal of Pharmacology*, 1914, **6**, 147–190.

Dale, H. H. Chemical Transmission of the effects of Nerve Impulses. *British Medical Bulletin*, 1934, **1**, 835–841.

Daniels, T. C., and Jorgensen, D. Physiochemical Properties in Relation to Biologic Action. In *Textbook of Organic Medicine and Pharmaceutical Chemistry*. C. O. Wilson, O. Gisvold, and R. F. Doerge Eds.). J. P. Lippincott, Philadelphia, 1971.

Davis, W. M. Day-Night Periodicity in Pentobarbital Response of Mice and the Influence of Socio-Psychological Conditions. *Expermentia*, 1962, **18**, 1–5.

DeLaTorre, J. C. Relative Penetration of L-Dopa and 5-Hydroxytryptophan Through the Brain Barrier Using Dimethyl Sulfoxide. *Experientia*, 1970, **26**, 1117–1118.

Del Castillo, J., and Katz, B. The Effect of Magnesium on the Activity of Motor Nerve Endings. *Journal of Physiology*, 1954, **124**, 553–559.

Denenberg, V. H., and Whimbey, A. E. Infantile Stimulation and Animal Husbandry: a Methodological Study. *Journal of Comparative and Physiological Psychology*, 1963, **56**, 877–878.

De Robertis, E. D. D. Submicroscopic Morphology of the Synapse. *International Review of Cytology*, 1959, **8**, 61–96.

De Robertis, E., and Vaz Ferreira, A. Submicroscopic Changes in Nerve Endings in the Adrenal Medulla after Stimulation of the Splanchnic Nerve. *Journal of Biophysics and Biochemical Cytology*, 1957, **3**, 611–614.

Dethier, V. G. Summation and Inhibition Following Contralateral Stimulation of the Tarsal Chemoreceptors of the Blowfly. *Biological Bulletin*, 1953, **105**, 257–268.

Dewey, W. L., Harris, L. S., and Kennedy, J. S. Some Pharmacological and Toxicological Effects of 1-trans-Δ^8 and 1-trans-Δ^9-Tetrahydrocannabinol in Laboratory Rats. *Archives Internationales de Pharmacodynamie et de Thérapie*, 1972, **196**, 133–145

Dews, P. B. The Measurement of the Influences of Drugs in Voluntary Activity in Mice. *British Journal of Pharmacology*, 1953, **8**, 46–48.

Dews, P. B. Studies on Behavior. IV Stimulant Actions of Methamphetamine. *Journal of Pharmacology*, 1958, **122**, 137–147.

Doluisio, J. T., and Swintosky, J. W. Biopharmaceutics. In *Remington's Pharmaceutic Sciences*. Mack Publishing Co., Easton, Pa., 1965.

Domek, N. S., Barlow, C. F., and Roth, L. J. An Ontogenetic Study of Phenobarbital-C[14] in Cat Brain. *Journal of Pharmacology and Experimental Therapeutics*, 1960, **130**, 285–293.

Domino, E. F. Antianxiety Drugs. In *Drill's Pharmacology in Medicine*. J. R. Dipalma (Ed.). McGraw-Hill, New York, 1971, pp. 489–498.

Driscoll, S. G., and Hsia, D. Y. The Development of Enzyme Systems During Early Infancy. *Pediatrics*, 1958, **22**, 785–845.

Eccles, J. C. *The Inhibitory pathways of the Central Nervous System*. Liverpool University Press, Liverpool, 1969.

Eccles, J. C., Schmidt, R., and Willis, W. D. Pharmacological Studies on Presynaptic Inhibition. *Journal of Physiology*, 1963, **168**, 500–530.

Edwards, A. L. *Experimental Design in Psychological Research*. Holt, Rinehart and Winston, New York, 1965.

Ehrenpreis, S., and Teller, D. N. Interaction of Drugs of Dependence with Receptors. In *Chemical and Biological Aspects of Drug Dependence*. S. J. Mulé and H. Brill (Eds.). CRC Press, Cleveland, 1972, pp. 177–217.

Ehrlich, P. Chemotherapeutics: Scientific Principles, Methods and Results. *Lancet*, **1913**(2), 445–451.

Elliott, H. C. *Textbook of Neuroanatomy*. J. P. Lippincott, Philadelphia, 1972.

Elliott, K. A. C., Swank, R. L., and Henderson, N. Effects of Anesthetics and Convulsants on Acetylcholine Content of Brain. *American Journal of Physiology*, 1950, **162**, 469–474.

Eriksson, K. Behavioral and Physiological Differences Among Rat Strains Specifically Selected for Their Alcohol Consumption. *Annals of the New York Academy of Sciences*, 1972, **197**, 32–41.

Essig, C. F. Barbiturates Withdrawal Convulsions in Decerebellate Dogs. *International Journal of Neuropharmacology*, 1964, **3**, 453–456.

Everett, N. B. *Functional Neuroanatomy*. Lea and Febiger, Philadelphia, 1971.

Fatt, P., and Katz, B. Some Observations on Biological Noise. *Nature*, 1950, **166**, 597–598.

Faulconer, A., and Bickford, R. G. *Electroencephalography in Anesthesiology*. Charles C Thomas, Springfield, Ill., 1960.

Feldberg, W. Present Views on the Mode of Action of Acetylcholine in the Central Nervous System. *Physiological Review*, 1945, **25**, 596–642.

Feldberg, W., and Sherwood, S. L. Injections of Drugs into the Lateral Ventricle of the Cat. *Journal of Physiology*, 1954, **123**, 148–167.

Ferguson, A., Henriksen, S., Cohen, H., Mitchell, G., Barachas, J., and Dement, W. "Hypersexuality" and Behavioral Changes in Cats Caused by Administraion of *p*-Chlorophenylalanine. *Science*, 1970, **168**, 499–501.

Ferguson, J. The Use of Chemical Potentials as Indices of Toxicity. *Proceedings of the Royal Society*, 1939, **127B**, 387–404.

Fischer, A. E., and Coury, J. N. Chemical Tracing of Neural Pathways Mediating the Thirst Drive. In *Thirst*. M. J. Wayner (Ed.). Pergamon Press, New York, 1964, 515–526.

Fox, A. L. The Relationship Between Chemical Constitution and Taste. *Proceedings of the National Academy of Sciences*, 1932, **18**, 115–121.

Fox, T. M. Strains and Species Variations in Pharmacological Responses. *International Symposium on Laboratory Animals*, 1966, **5**, 133–148.

Frazier, D. T., Narahashi, T., and Yamada, M. The Site of Action and Active Form of Local Anesthetics. II. Experiments with Quaternary Compounds. *Journal of Pharmacology and Experimental Therapeutics*, 1970, **171**, 45–51.

Friede, R. L. *Topographic Brain Chemistry*. Academic Press, New York, 1966.

Friedman, M. J., Jaffe, J. H., and Sharpless, S. K. Central Nervous System Supersensitivity to Pilocarpine after Withdrawal of Chronically Administered Scopolamine. *Journal of Pharmacology and Experimental Therapeutics*, 1969, **167**, 45–55.

Fuller, J. L. Pharmacogenetics. In *Principles of Psychopharmacology*. W. G. Clark and J. del Guidice (Eds.). Academic Press, New York, 1970, 337–342.

Fuortes, M. G. R., and Nelson, P. G. Strychnine: Its Action on Spinal Motoneurons of Cats. *Science*, 1963, **140**, 806–808.

Furchgott, R. F. The Pharmacology of Vascular Smooth Muscle. *Pharmacological Review*, 1955, **7**, 183–265.

Furchgott, R. F. The Classification of Adrenoreceptors. In *Catecholamines*. H. Blaschko and E. Muscholl (Eds.). Springer-Verlag, New York, 1972, pp. 283–335.

Gaddum, J. H. Methods of Biological Assay Depending on a Quantal Response. *Medical Research Council, Special Report Series*, No. 183, London, 1933.

Gaddum, J. H. *Pharmacology*. Oxford University Press, London, 1959.

Gaddum, J. H., and Hameed, K. A. Drugs Which Antagonize 5-Hydroxytryptamine. *British Journal of Pharmacology*, 1954, **9**, 240–248.

Gardiner, J. E. The Inhibition of Acetylcholine in Brain by a Hemicholinum. *Biochemical Journal*, 1961, **81**, 297–303.

Gawienowski, A. M., and Hodgen, G. D. Homosexual Activity in Male Rats after *p*-Chlorophenylalanine: Effect of Hypophesectomy and Testosterone. *Physiology and Behavior*, 1971, **7**, 551–555.

Gay, H. Nuclear Control of the Cell. *Scientific American*, 1960, **202**, 126–136.

Gebhart, G. G., Sherman, A. D., and Mitchell, C. L. The Influence of Learning on Morphine Analgesia and Tolerance Development in Rats Tested on the Hot Plate. *Psychopharmacologia*, 1971, **22**, 295–304.

Gessa, G. L., Tagliamonte, A., Tagliamonte, P., and Brodie, B. B. Essential Role of Testosterone in the Sexual Stimulation Induced by *p*-Chlorophenylalanine in Male Animals. *Nature*, 1970, **227**, 616–617.

Gibaldi, M. *Introduction to Biopharmaceutics*. Lea and Febiger, Philadelphia, 1971.

Goldbaum, L. R., and Smith, P. K. The Interaction of Barbiturates with Serum Albumin and Its Possible Relation to Their Disposition and Pharmacological Actions. *Journal of Pharmacology and Experimetal Therapeutics*, 1954, **111**, 197–209.

Goldberg, N. D., and Shideman, F. E. Species Differences in the Cardia Effects of a Monoamine Oxidase Inhibitor. *Journal of Pharmacology and Experimental Therapeutics*, 1963, **136**, 142–151.

Goldberg, S. R., Hoffmeister, F., and Schlichting, U. U. Morphine Antagonists: Modification of Behavioral Effects by Morphine Dependence. In *Drug Addiction*: I. *Experimental Pharmacology*. J. M. Singh, L. Miller, and H. Lal (Eds.). Future Publishing Co., Mt. Kisco, N.Y., 1972.

Goldstein, A. The Interaction of Drugs and Plasma Proteins. *Pharmacological Review*, 1949, **1**, 102–165.

Goldstein, A., Aronow, L., and Kalman, S. *Principles of Drug Action*. Harper and Row, New York, 1969.

Goldstein, B., and Goldstein, A. Possible Role of Enzyme Inhibition and Repression in Drug Tolerance and Addiction. *Biochemical Pharmacology*, 1961, **8**, 48.

Goodman, L. S., and Gilman, A. *The Pharmacological Basis of Therapeutics*. Macmillan, New York, 1970.

Grahame-Smith, D. G. Tryptophan Hydroxylation in Brain. *Biochemical and Biophysical Research Communications*, 1964, **16**, 586–593 .(*a*)

Grahame-Smith, D. G. The Enzymatic Conversion of Tryptophan into 5-Hydroxytryptophan by Isolated Brain Tissue. *Biochemical Journal*, 1964, **92**, 52P. (*b*)

Grossman, S. P. Eating or Drinking Elicited by Direct Adrenergic of Cholinergic Stimulation of Hypothalamus. *Science*, 1960, **132**, 301–302.

Grossman, S. P. Direct Adrenergic and Cholinergic Stimulation of Hypothalamic Mechanisms. *American Journal of Physiology*, 1962, **202**, 872–882. (*a*)

Grossman, S. P. Effects of Adrenergic and Cholinergic Blocking Agents on Hypothalamic Mechanisms. *American Journal of Physiology*, 1962, **202**, 1230–1236. (*b*)

Haase, H. J., and Janssen, P. A. J. The Action of Neuroleptic Drugs. Year Book Medical Publishers, Chicago, 1965.

Halberg, F. Chronobiology. *Annual Review of Physiology*, 1969, **31**, 675–725.

Hald, J. E., and Jacobsen, E. The Formation of Acetaldehyde in the Organism after Injection of Antabuse (Tetraethylthiuramdisulphide) and Alcohol. *Acta Pharmacologia et Toxicologia*, 1948, **4**, 305–310.

Halton, P., and Perry, W. L. M. On the Transmitter Responsible for Antidromic Vasodilation in the Rabbit's Ear. *Journal of Physiology*, 1951, **114**, 240–251.

Hanig, J. P., Morrison, J. M., and Krop, S. Influence of Blood-Brain Permeability to Catecholamines by Dimethyl Sulfoxide in the Neonatal Chick. *Journal of Pharmacy and Pharmacology*, 1971, **23**, 386–387.

Hanig, J. P., Morrison, J. M., and Krop, S. Ethanol Enhancement of Blood-Brain Barrier Permeability to Catecholamines in Chicks. *European Journal of Pharmacology*, 1972, **18**, 79–82.

Hartshorn, E. A. *Handbook of Drug Interactions*. D. E. Franke, Cincinnati, 1970.

Haus, E., and Halberg, F. Circannual Rhythm in Level and Timing of Serum Corticosterone in Standardized Inbred Mature C^1-Mice. *Environmental Research*, 1970, **3**, 81–106.

Hazelton, L. W., and Hellerman, R. C. The Influence of Vehicles on the Actions of Drugs. *Journal of the American Pharmaceutical Association*, 1946, **35**, 161–168.

Hebb, C. O. Biochemical Evidence for the Neural Functions of Acetylcholine. *Physiological Review*, 1957, **37**, 196–220.

Hebb, C. O., and Silver, A. Choline Acetylase in the Central Nervous System of Man and Some Other Mammals. *Journal of Physiology*, 1956, **134**, 718–728.

Hebb, D. O. *The Organization of Behavior*. John Wiley, New York, 1949.

Hebb, D. O. Drives and the C.N.S. (Conceptual Nervous System). *Psychological Review*, 1955, **62**, 243–254.

Hebb, D. O. *A Textbook of Psychology*. W. B. Saunders, Philadelphia, 1966.

Hewitt, H. B. A Sensitive Method for the Assay of Androgens Based on the Power to Alter Reactions of the Mouse Kidney to Chloroform. *Journal of Endocrinology*, 1957, **14**, 394–399.

Hill, H. E., Belleville, R. E., and Wikler, A. Motivational Determinants in Modification of Behavior by Morphine and Pentobarbital. *American Medical Association Archives of Neurology and Psychiatry*, 1957, **77**, 28–35.

Hodgkin, A. L. Ionic Movements and Electrical Activity in Giant Nerve Fibres. *Proceedings of the Royal Society*, 1958, **148**, 1–37.

Hodgkin, A. L., and Keynes, R. D. Active Transport of Cations in Giant Axons for *Sepia* and *Loligo*. *Journal of Physiology*, 1955, **128**, 28–60.

Hogben, C. A. M., Schanker, L. S., Tocco, D. J., and Brodie, B. B. Absorption of Drugs from the Stomach. II. The Human. *Journal of Pharmacology and Experimental Therapeutics*, 1957, **120**, 540–545.

Hollister, L. E., Matzenbecker, F. P., and Degan, R. O. Withdrawal Reactions for Chlordiazepoxide ("Librium"). *Psychopharmacologia*, 1961, **2**, 63–68.

Holter, H. Pinocytosis. *International Review of Cytology*, 1959, **8**, 481–504.

Hornykiewicz, O. Dopamine and Brain Function. *Pharmacological Review*, 1966, **18**, 925–563.

Hucker, H. B. Species Differences in Drug Metabolism. *Annual Review of Pharmacology*, 1970, **10**, 99–118.

Hug, C. C. Characteristics and Theories Related to Acute and Chronic Tolerance Development. In *Chemical and Biological Aspects of Drug Dependence*. S. J. Mulé and H. Brill (Eds.). CRC Press, Cleveland, 1972, pp. 307–358.

Irwin, S. Factors Influencing Sensitivity to Stimulant and Depressant Drugs Affecting (A) Locomotor and (B) Conditioned Avoidance Behavior in Animals. In *The Dynamics of Psychiatric Drug Therapy*. G. J. Sarwer-Fomer (Ed.). Charles C Thomas, Springfield, Ill., 1960, pp. 5–22.

Irwin, S., Slabok, M., and Thomas, G. Individual Differences: I. Correlation between Locomotor Activity and Sensitivity to Stimulant and Depressant Drugs. *Journal of Pharmacology and Experimental Therapeutics*, 1958, **123**, 206–211.

Isbell, H., Wolbach, A. B., Wikler, A., and Miner, E. J. Cross Tolerance between LSD and Psilocybin. *Psychopharmacologia*, 1961, **2**, 147–159.

Israel, Y., Kalant, H., and LeBlanc, E. Effects of Lower Alcohols on Potassium Transport and Microsomal Adenosine-Triphosphate Activity of Rat Cerebral Cortex. *Biochemical Journal*, 1966, **100**, 27–33.

Jacob, J. The Influence of Variation in Species and Strains of Experimental Animals on Drug Responses. In *Importance of Fundamental Principles in Drug Evaluation*. D. H. Tedeschi and R. E. Tedeschi (Eds.). Raven Press, New York, 1969, pp. 383–405.

Jacobson, E. *Progressive Relaxation*. University of Chicago Press, Chicago, 1938.

Jaffe, J. H., and Sharpless, S. K. Pharmacological Denervation Supersensitivity in the Central Nervous System: A Theory of Physical Dependence. In *Addictive States*. A. Wikler (Ed.). Williams and Wilkins, Baltimore, 1968, pp.226–246.

Janssen, P. A. J. The Pharmacology of Haloperidol. *International Journal of Neuropsychiatry*, 1967, **3**, Supplement 1.

Jarvik, M. E. Drug Used in the Treatment of Psychiatric Disorders. In *The Pharmacological Basis of Therapeutics*. L. S. Goodman and A. Gilman (Eds.). Macmillan ,New York, 1970, pp. 151–203.

Jasper, H. H. Electroencephalography. In *Epilepsy and Cerebral Localization*. W. Penfield and T. C. Erickson (Eds.). Charles C Thomas, Springfield, Ill., 1941.

Kalant, H., LeBlanc, A. E., and Gibbins, R. J. Tolerance to, and Dependence on Some Non-Opiate Psychotropic Drugs. *Pharmacological Review*, 1971, **23**, 135–191.

Kalow, W. *Pharmacogenetics*. W. B. Saunders, Philadelphia, 1962.

Kandel, E. R., and Spencer, W. A. Cellular Neurophysiological Approaches in the Study of Learning. *Physiological Review*, 1968, **48**, 65–134.

Kato, R., Chiesara, E., and Frontino, G. Influence of Sex Differences on the Pharmacological Actions and Metabolism of Some Drugs. *Biochemical Pharmacology*, 1962, **11**, 221–227.

Kelleher, R. T., and Morse, W. H. Determinants of the Specificity of Behavioral Effects of Drugs. *Ergebnisse der Physiologie*, 1968, **60**, 1–56.

Kerr, F. W. L., and Pozuelo, J. Suppression of Physical Dependence and Induction of Hypersensitivity to Morphine by Stereotaxic Hypothalamic Lesions in Addicted Rats. *Mayo Clinic Proceedings*, 1971, **46**, 653–665.

Key, B. J., and Marley, E. The Effect of the Sympathomimetic Amines on Behavior and Electrocortical Activity of the Chicken. *Electroencephalography and Clinical Neurophysiology*, 1962, **14**, 90–105.

Khavari, K. A., and Russel, R. W. Acquisition, Retention, and Extinction under Conditions of Water Deprivation and of Central Cholinergic Stimulation. *Journal of Comparative and Physiological Psychology*, 1966, **61**, 339–345.

Killam, E. K. Pharmacology of the Reticular Formation. In *Psychopharmacology*. D. E. Efron (Ed.). Washington, 1968, 411–445.

King, A., and Little, J. C. Thiopental Treatment of the Phobic-Anxiety-Depersonalization Syndrome. *Proceedings of the Royal Society of Medicine*, 1959, **52**, 595–596.

Kleeman, C. R., Davson, H., and Levin, E. Urea Transport in the Central Nervous System. *American Journal of Physiology*, 1962, **203**, 739–747.

Knoll, J. Motimeter, A New Sensitive Apparatus for the Quantitative Measure of Hypermotility Caused by Psychostimulants. *Archives Internationales de Pharmacodynamie et de Thérapie*, 1961, **130**, 141–154.

Knox, W. E., Auerbach, V. H., and Lin, E. C. C. Enzymatic and Metabolic Adaptations in Animals. *Physiological Review*, 1956, **36**, 164–254.

Koelle, G. B. A New General Concept of the Neurohumoral Functions of Acetylcholine and Acetylcholinesterase. *Journal of Pharmacy and Pharmacology*, 1962, **14**, 65–90.

Kopin, I. J. False Adrenergic Transmitters. In *Perspectives in Neuropharmacology*. S. H. Snyder (Ed.). Oxford University Press, New York, 1972.

Koppanyi, T., and Avery, M. A. Species Differences and the Chemical Trial of New Drugs: A Review. *Clinical Pharmacology and Therapy*, 1966, 7, 250–270.

Kornetsky, C. Psychoactive Drugs in the Immature Organism. *Psychopharmacologia*, 1970, **17**, 105–136.

Koshland, D. E. Enzyme Flexibility and Enzyme Action. *Journal of Cellular and Comparative Physiology*, 1959, **45**, 245–258.

Kretchmer, N. Enzymatic Patterns During Development. An Approach to a Biochemical Definition of Immaturity. *Pediatrics*, 1959, **23**, 606–617.

Krnjević, K., and Phillis, J. W. Acetylcholine-Sensitive Cells in the Cerebral Cortex. *Journal of Physiology*, 1963, **166**, 296–327. (*a*)

Krnjević, K., and Phillis, J. W. Pharmacological Properties of Acetylcholine-Sensitive Cells in the Cerebral Cortex. *Journal of Physiology*, 1963, **166**, 328–350. (*b*)

Krnjević, K., and Schwartz, S. Some Properties of Unresponsive Cells in the Cerebral Cortex. *Experimental Brain Research*, 1967, **3**, 306–319.

Krnjević, K., Punain, R., and Renaud, L. The Mechanism of Excitation by Acetylcholine in the Cerebral Cortex. *Journal of Physiology*, 1971, **215**, 247–268.

Kuhar, M. J., Pert, C. B., and Snyder, S. H. Regional Distribution of Opiate Receptor Binding in Monkey and Human Brain. *Nature*, 1973, **245**, 447–450.

Kulkarni, A., and Shideman, F. E. Sensitivities of the Brains of Infant and Adult Rats to the Catecholamine-Depleting Actions of Reserpine and Tetrabenazine. *Journal of Pharmacology and Experimental Therapeutics*, 1966, **153**, 428–433.

Kuntzman, R., Shore, P. A., Bogdanski, D. F., and Brodie, B. B. Microanalytical Procedures for Fluorometric Assay of Brain Dopa, 5-HTP Decarboxylase, Norepinephrine, and Serotonin; and a Detailed Mapping of Decarboxylase Activity in the Brain. *Journal of Neurochemistry*, 1961, **6**, 226–232.

LaDu, B. N. Genetic Factors Modifying Drug Metabolism and Drug Responses. In *Fundamentals of Drug Metabolism and Drug Disposition*. B. N. LaDu, H. G. Mandel, and E. L. Way (Eds.). Williams and Wilkins, Baltimore, 1971.

Lajtha, A. The Development of the Blood-Brain Barrier. *Journal of Neurochemistry*, 1957, **1**, 228–233.

Langley, J. N. On Nerve Endings and on Special Excitable Substances in Cells. *Proceedings of the Royal Society*, 1906, **78B**, 170–194.

Lashley, K. In Search of the Engram. *Symposium of the Society of Experimental Biology*, 1950, **4**, 454–482.

Laverty, R., Sharman, D. F., and Vogt, M. Action of 2,4,5-Trihydroxyphenylethylamine on the Storage and Release of Noradrenaline. *British Journal of Pharmacology*, 1965, **24**, 549–560.

Lee, C. Comparative Pharmacologic Responses to Antihistamines in Newborn and Young Rats. *Toxicology and Applied Pharmacology*, 1966, **8**, 210–217.

Levitt, R. A., and Fisher, A. E. Anticholinergic Blockage of Centrally Induced Thirst. *Science*, 1966, **154**, 520–522.

Lewis, W. H. Pinocytosis by Malignant Cells. *American Journal of Cancer*, 1937, **29**, 666–679.

Lindsay, H. A., and Kullman, V. S. Pentobarbital Sodium: Variation in Toxicity. *Science*, 1966, **151**, 576–577.

Lindsley, D. B. Emotion. In *Handbook of Experimental Psychology*. S. S. Stevens (Ed.). John Wiley, New York, 1951.

Lloyd, S., and Pickford, M. An Examination of Certain Factors which Might or Do, Affect the Vascular Response to Oxytocin. *Journal of Physiology*, 1967, **193**, 547–569.

Loewi, O. Über humorale Übertragbarkeit der Herznervenwirkung. I. *Pflügers Archiv für die Gesante Physiologie*, 1921, **189**, 239–242.

Lomax, P., and Kirkpatrick, W. E. The Effect of *N*-Allylnormorphine on the Development of Acute Tolerance to the Analgesic and Hypothermic Effects of Morphine in the Rat. *Medical Pharmacology*, 1967, **16**, 165–170.

Loomis, T. A. *Essentials of Toxicology*. Lea and Febiger, Philadelphia, 1968.

Lutsch, E. F., and Morris, R. W. Circadian Periodicity in Susceptibility to Lidocaine Hydrochloride. *Science*, 1967, **156**, 100–102.

MacIntosh, F. C. Formation, Storage, and Release of Acetylcholine at Nerve Endings. *Canadian Journal of Biochemistry and Physiology*, 1959, **37**, 343–356.

MacIntosh, F. C. Synthesis and Storage of Acetylcholine in Nervous Tissue. *Canadian Journal of Biochemistry and Physiology*, 1963 **41**, 2555–2571.

MacIntosh, F. C., Birks, R. I., and Sastry, P. B. Pharmacological Inhibition of Acetylcholine Synthesis. *Nature*, 1956, **178**, 1181.

MacIntosh, F. C., Birks, R. I., and Sastry, P. B. Mode of Action of an Inhibitor of Acetylcholine Synthesis. *Neurology*, 1958, **8**, 90–91.

MacLean, P. D. Chemical and Electrical Stimulation of Hippocampus in Unrestrained Animals. I. Methods and Electroencepahlographic Findings. *Archives of Neurology*, 1957, **78**, 113–127.

Marazzi, A. S., Hart, E. R., and Cohn, V. H. Pharmacology of the Nervous System. *Progress in Neurology and Psychiatry*, 1956, **11**, 565–594

Mark, L. C., Burns, J. J., and Brand, L., Campomanes, C. I., Trousof, N., Popper, E. M., and Brodie, B. B. The passage of Thiobarbiturates and their Oxygen Analogs into the Brain. *Journal of Pharmacology and Experimental Therapeutics*, 1958, **123**, 70–73.

Marsh, D. F. *Outline of Pharmacology*. Charles C Thomas, Springfield, Ill., 1951.

Marsland, D. The Site of Narcosis in a Cell, The Action of a Series of Parrafin Oils on Amoebia Dubia. *Journal of Cellular and Comparative Physiology*, 1394, **4**, 9–33.

Martin, W. R. Pharmacological Redundancy as an Adaptive Mechanism in the Central Nervous System. *Federation Proceedints*, 1970, **29**, 13–18.

Martin, W. R., and Eades, C. G. Pharmacological Studies of Spinal Cord Adrenergic and Cholinergic Mechanisms and their Relations to Physical Dependence on Morphine. *Psychopharmacologia*, 1967, **11**, 195–223.

Masserman, J. H. Drugs, Brain and Behavior. An Experimental Approach to Experimental Psychoses. *Journal of Neuropsychiatry*, 1962, **3**, S104–S113.

Matthews, B. H. C. The Response of a Single End Organ. *Journal of Physiology*, 1931, **71**, 64–110.

Mayer, S. E., and Bain, J. A. Localization of the Hematoencephalic Barrier with Fluorescent Quaternary Acridones. *Journal of Pharmacology and Experimental Therapeutics*, 1956, **118**, 17–25.

Mayer, S., Maickel, R. P., and Brodie, B. B. Kinetics of Penetration of Drugs and Other Foreign Compounds into Cerebrospinal Fluid and Brain. *Journal of Pharmacology and Experimental Therapeutics*, 1959, **127**, 205–211.

Maynert, E. W. Sedatives and Hypnotics. II. Barbiturates. In *Drill's Pharmacology in Medicine*. J. R. Dipalma (Ed.). McGraw-Hill, New York, 1971.

McCarthy, L. E., and Borrison, H. L. Volumetric Compartmentalization of the Cranial Cerebrospinal Fluid System Determined Radiographically in the Cat. *Anatomical Record*, 1966, **155**, 305–314.

McCarthy, L. E., and Borrison, H. L. Ventricular Cerebrospinal Fluid Dynamics Examined Radiographically in the Cat. *Experimental Neurology*, 1967, **17**, 57–64.

McClearn, G. E., and Rodgers, D. A. Differences in Alcohol Preferences among Inbred Strains of Mice. *Quarterly Journal of Studies on Alcohol*, 1959, **20**, 691–695.

McLennan, H. *Synaptic Transmission*. W. B. Saunders, Philadelphia, 1970.

Meier, H. *Experimental Pharmacogenetics*. Academic Press, New York, 1963.

Mennear, J. H., and Rudzik, A. D. The Effects of Alpha and Beta Adrenergic Blockade in the Lethality of Amphetamine in Aggregated Mice. *Life Sciences*, 1965, **4**, 1425–1432.

Meyer, H. Zur Theorie der Alkonarkose. *Archiv für Experimentelle Pathologie und Pharmakologie*, 1901, **46**, 338–346.

Meyer, K. H. Contributions to the Theory of Narcosis. *Transactions of the Faraday Society*, 1937, **33**, 1062–1068.

Meyer, K. H., and Hemmi, H. Beiträge zur Theorie der Narkose. III. *Biochemische Zeitschrift*, 1935, **277**, 39–71.

Miller, N. E. Effects of Drugs on Motivation: The Value of Using a Variety of Measures. *Annals of the New York Academy of Sciences*, 1956, **65**, 318–333.

Miller, N., Gottesman, K., and Emery, N. Dose Response to Carbacol and Norepinephrine in Rat Hypothalamus. *American Journal of Physiology*, 1964, **206**, 1384–1388.

Mirsky, A. F., and Kornetsky, C. The Effect of Centrally-acting Drugs on Attention. In *Psychopharmacology*. D. H. Efron (Ed.). Washington, 1968, pp. 91–104.

Mitchell, J. F. The Spontaneous and Evoked Release of Acetylcholine from the Cerebral Cortex. *Journal of Physiology*, 1963, **165**, 98–116.

Molitor, H. A. A Comparative Study of the Effects of Five Choline Compounds Used in Therapeutics. *Journal of Pharmacology and Experimental Therapeutics*, 1937, **58**, 337–360.

Moser, K., Papenberg, J., and Wartburg, J. P. Heterogenität und Organerteilung der Alkoholdehydrogenase bei verschiedenen Spezies. *Enzymologia Biologica Clinica*, 1968, **9**, 447–458.

Munkvad, I., Pakkenberg, H., and Randrup, A. Aminergic Systems in Basal Ganglia Associated with Stereotyped Hyperactive Behavior and Catelepsy. *Brain, Behavior, and Evolution*, 1968, **1**, 89–100.

Murphree, H. B. Narcotic Analgesics. I. Opium Alkaloids. In *Drill's Pharmacology in Medicine*, J. R. Diplama (Ed.). McGraw-Hill, New York, 1971, pp. 324–349.

Muscholl, E. Cholinomimetic Drugs and Release of the Adrenergic Transmitter. In *New Aspects of Storage and Release Mechanisms of Catecholamines*. H. J. Schumann and G. Kroneberg (Eds.). Springer-Verlag, New York, 1970, pp. 168–186.

Myers, R. D. Modification of Drinking Patterns by Chronic Intracranial Chemical Infusion. In *Thirst*. M. J. Wayner (Ed.). Pergamon Press, New York, 1964, pp. 533–552.

Myers, R. D. Chemical Mechanisms in the Hypothalamus Mediating Eating and Drinking in the Monkey. *Annals of the New York Academy of Sciences*, 1969, **157**, 918–933.

Nachmansohn, D. *Chemical and Molecular Basis of Nerve Activity*. Academic Press, New York, 1959.

Nagatsu, R., Levitt, M., and Udenfriend, S. Conversion of L-Tyrosine to 3,4-Dihydroxyphenylalanine by Cell-Free Preparations of Brain and Sympathetically Innervated Tissues. *Biochemistry and Biophysics Research Communications*, 1964, **14**, 543–549.

Narahashi, T., Anderson, N. C., and Moore, J. W. Comparison of Tetrodotoxin and Procaine in Internally Perfused Squid Giant Axons. *Journal of General Physiology*, 1967, **50**, 1413–1428.

Narahashi, R., Frazier, D. T., and Yamada, M. The Site of Action and Active Form of Local Anaesthetics. I. Theory and pH Experiments with Tertiary Compounds. *Journal of Pharmacology and Experimental Therapeuctics*, 1970, **171**, 32–44.

Nayler, W. G. Seasonal Variation in Cardiac Phosphorylase A Activity. *Life Sciences*, 1968, **7**, 295–299.

Neal, M., Hemisworth, B. A., and Mitchell, J. F. The Excitation of Central Cholinergic Mechanisms by Stimulation of the Auditory Pathway. *Life Sciences*, 1968, **7**, 757–763.

Nickerson, M. Receptor Occupancy and Tissue Response. *Nature*, 1956, **178**, 697–687.

Nora, J. J., Smith, W. D., and Cameron, J. R. The Route of insulin administration in the Management of Diabetes Mellitus. *Journal of Pediatrics*, 1964, **64**, 547–551.

Nyhan, W. L. Toxicity of Drugs in the Neonatal Period. *Journal of Pediatrics*, 1961, **59**, 1–20.

Olds, J., and Milner, P. J. Positive Reinforcement Produced by Electrical Stimulation of Septal Area and Other Regions of Rat Brain. *Journal of Comparative and Physiological Psychology*, 1954, **47**, 419–427.

Olds, J., and Travis, R. P. Effects of Chlorpromazine, Meprobamate, Pentobarbital, and Morphine on Self-Stimulation. *Journal of Pharmacology and Experimental Therapeutics*, 1960, **128**, 397–404.

Osmond, H. A Review of the Chemical Effects of Psychotomimetic Agents. *Annals of the New York Academy of Sciences*, 1957, **66**, 418–434.

Oster, G. Phosphenes. *Scientific American*, 1970, **222**, 82–87.

Oswald, I., and Priest, R. G. Five Weeks to Escape the Sleeping-Pill Habit. *British Medical Journal*, 1965, **2**, 1093–1096.

Overton, E. *Studien über die Narkose Zugleich ein Beitrag zur allgemeinen Pharmakologie*. Verlag von Gustav Fisher, Jena, 1901.

Papez, J. W. A Proposed Mechanism of Emotion. *Archives of Neurology and Psychiatry*, 1937, **38**, 725–743.

Papez, J. W. The Visceral Brain, Its Components and Connections. In *Reticular Formation of the Brain*. H. H. Jasper (Ed.). Little, Brown, Boston, 1959.

Paton, W. D. M. A Theory of Drug Action Based on the Rate of Drug-Receptor Combination. *Proceedings of the Royal Society*, 1961, **154B**, 21–69.

Pert, C. B., and Snyder, S. H. Opiate Receptor: Demonstration in Nervous Tissue. *Science*, 1973, **79**, 1011–1014.

Pert, C. B., Pasternak, G., and Snyder, S. H. Opiate Agonists and Antagonists Discriminated by Receptor Binding in Brain, *Science*, 1973, **182**,1359–1361.

Philippu, A. Release of Catecholamines from the Hypothalamus by Drugs and Electrical Stimulation. In *New Aspects of Storage and Release Mechanisms of Catecholamines*. H. J. Schumann and G. Kroneberg (Eds.). Springer-Verlag, New York, 1970, pp. 258–267.

Phillips, R. M., Miya, T. S., and Yin, G. K. W. Studies on the Mechanism of Meprobamate Tolerance in the Rat. *Journal of Pharmacology and Experimental Therapeutics*, 1962, **135**, 223–229.

Phillis, J. W. *The Pharmacology of Synapses*. Pergamon Press, London, 1970.

Plummer, A. J., Earl, A., Schneider, J. A., Trapold, J., and Barrett, W. Pharmacology of Rauwolfia Alkaloids Including Reserpine. *Annals of the New York Academy of Sciences*, 1954, **59**, 8–21.

Porter, C. C., Totero, J. A., and Stone, C. A. Effect of 6-Hydroxydopamine and Some Other Compounds on the Concentration of Norepinephrine in the Hearts of Mice. *Journal of Pharmacology and Experimental Therapeutics*, 1963, **140**, 308–316.

Poschel, B. P. H., and Ninteman, F. W. Norepinephrine: A Possibel Excitatory Neurohormone of the Reward System. *Life Sciences*, 1963, **2**, 782–788.

Porschel, B. P. H., and Ninteman, F. W. Excitatory (Antidepressant?) Effects of Monoamine Oxidase Inhibitors on the Reward System of the Brain. *Life Sciences*, 1964, **3**, 903–910.

Potter, L. T., and Molinoff, P. B. Isolation of Cholinergic Receptor Proteins. In *Persepctives in Neuropharmacology*. S. H. Snyder (Ed.). Oxford University Press, New York, 1972, pp. 9–42.

Przbyla, A. C., and Wang, S. C. Locus of Central Depressant Action of Diazepam. *Journal of Pharmacology and Experimental Therapeutics*, 1968, **163**, 439–447.

Quastel, J. H. Effects of Neurotropic Drugs on Brain Metabolism in Vitro. In *Molecular Basis of Some Aspects of Mental Activity*. O. Walaas (Ed.). Academic Press, New York, 1967, Vol. 2, pp. 19–37.

Quinn, G. P., Axelrod, J., and Brodie, B. B. Species, Strain and Sex Differences in Metabolism of Hexobarbitone, Amidopyrine, Antipyrine, and Aniline. *Biochemical Pharmacology*, 1958, **1**, 152–159.

Radzialowski, F. M., and Bousquet, W. F. Daily Rhythmic Variation in Hepatic Drug Metabolism in the Rat and Mouse. *Journal of Pharmacology and Experimental Therapeutics*, 1968, **163**, 229–238.

Ramón y Cajal, S. *Histologie du système nerveux de l'homme et des vertébrés*. Consejo Superior de Investigaciones Cientificas, Madrid, 1911.

Randall, L. O., Heise, G. A., and Schaller, W. Pharmacological and Chemical Studies on Valium, a New Psychotherapeutic Agent of the Benzodiazepine Class. *Current Therapeutic Research*, 1961, **3**, 405–425.

Rang, H. P., and Ritter, J. M. A New Kind of Drug Antagonism: Evidence that Agonists Cause a Molecular Change in Acetylcholine Receptors. *Molecular Pharmacology*, 1969, **5**, 394–411.

Rapoport, M. I., Feigin, R. D., Bruton, R. D., and Beisil, W. R. Circadian Rhythm for Tryptophan Pyrrolase Activity and its Circulating Substrate. *Science*, 1966, **153**, 1642–1644.

Ray, O. S. *Drugs, Society and Human Behavior*. C. V. Mosby, St. Louis, 1972.

Rech, R. H. The Relevance of Experiments Involving Injection of Drugs into the Brain. In *Importance of Fundamental Principles in Drug Evaluation*. D. H. Tedeschi and R. E. Tedeschi (Eds.). Raven Press, New York, 1968.

Rech, R. H., and Domino, E. F. Observations on Injections of Drugs into the Brain Substance. *Archives Internationales de Pharmacodynamie et de Thérapie*, 1959, **121**, 429–442.

Reed, J. A Study of the Alcoholic Consumption and Amino Acid Excretion Patterns of Rats of Different Inbred Strains. *University of Texas Publications*, 1951, **5109**, 144–149.

Reinberg, A., and Halberg, F. Circadian Chronopharmacology. *Annual Review of Pharmacology*, 1971, **11**, 455–492.

Reis, D. J., Corvelli, A., and Conners, J. Circadian and Ultradian Rhythms of Serotonin in Cat Brain. *Journal of Pharmacology and Experimental Therapeutics*, 1969, **167**, 328–333.

Richter, C. P. *Biological Clocks in Medicine and Psychiatry*. Charles C Thomas, Springfield, Ill., 1965.

Richter, D., and Crossland, J. Variation in Acetylcholine Content of the Brain with Physiological State. *American Journal of Physiology*, 1949, **159**, 247–255.

Ritchie, J. M., and Armett, C. J. On the Role of Acetylcholine in Mammalian Non-myelinated Nerve Fibres. *Journal of Pharmacology*, 1963, **139**, 201–207.

Roach, M. K. The Effect of Ethanol in the Synthesis of Amino Acids from Glucose in the Hamster Brain. *Life Sciences*, 1970, **9**, 437–441.

Roberts, M. H. T., and Straughan, D. W. Excitation and Depression of Cortical Neurones by 5-Hydroxytryptamine. *Journal of Physiology*, 1967, **193**, 269–294.

Robinson, G. A., Dobbs, J. W., and Sutherland, E. W. On the Nature of Receptor Sites for Biogenic Amines. In *Biogenic Amines as Physiological Regulators*. J. J. Blum Ed.). Prentice-Hall, Englewood Cliffs, New Jersey, 1970.

Rosen, H., Blumenthal, A., Panascvich, R., and McCallum, J. Dimethyl Sulfoxide (DMSO) as a Solvent in Acute Toxicity Determination. *Proceedings of the Society for Experimental Biology and Medicine*, 1965, **120**, 511–514.

Roth, L. J., Schoolas, J. C., and Barlow, C. F. Sulphur-35 Labelled Acetazolamide in Cat Brain. *Journal of Pharmacology and Experimental Therapeutics*, 1959, **125**, 128–136.

Rushton, R., and Steinberg, H. Modification of Behavioral Effects of Drugs by Past Experience. In *Animal Behavior and Drug Action*. A. V. S. de Reuck and J. Knight (Eds.) Little, Brown, Boston, 1964.

Schanker, L. S. Passage of Drugs Across Body Membranes. *Pharmacological Review*, 1962, **14**, 501–530.

Schanker, L. S. Physiological Transport of Drugs. *Advances in Drug Research*, 1964, **1**, 72–106.

Schanker, L. S., Shore, P. A., Brodie, B. B., and Hogben, C. A. M. Absorption of Drugs From the Stomach. I. The Rat. *Journal of Pharmacology and Experimental Therapeutics*, 1957, **120**, 528–539.

Scheving, L. E., Harrison, W. H., Gordon, P., and Pauly, J. E. Daily Fluctuations (Circadian and Ultradian) in Biogenic Amines of the Rat Brain. *American Journal of Physiology*, 1968, **214**, 166–173.

Schriftman, H., and Kondritzer, A. A. Absorption of Atropine from Muscle. *American Journal of Physiology*, 1957, **191**, 591–594.

Schuster, C. R. Psychological Approaches to Opiate Dependence and Self-Administration by Laboratory Animals. *Federation Proceedings*, 1970, **29**, 2–5.

Schuster, C. R., and Thompson, R. Self Administration of and Behavioral Dependence on Drugs. *Annual Review of Pharmacology*, 1969, **9**, 483–502.

Seeman, P. The Membrane Actions of Anesthetics and Tranquilizers. *Pharmacological Review*, 1972, **24**, 583–655.

Seevers, H. H., and Deneau, H. A. Physiological Aspects of Tolerance and Physical Dependence. In *Physiological Pharmacology*. W. S. Root and F. G. Hofmann (Eds.). Academic Press, New York, 1963, Vol. I. pp. 565–640.

Shanes, A. M. Electrochemical Aspects of Physiological and Pharmacological Action in Excitable Cells. I. The Resting Cell and Its Alteration by Extrinsic Factors. *Pharmacological Review*, 1958, **10**, 59–164.

Sharpless, S. K. Hypnotics and Sedatives. In *The Pharmacological Basis of Therapeutics*. L. S. Goodman and A. Gilman (Eds.). Macmillan, New York, 1970.

Shemano, I., and Nickerson, M. Effect of Ambient Temperature on Thermal Response to Drugs. *Canadian Journal of Physiology*, 1958, **36**, 1243–1249.

Shepherd, M. M., Lader, M., and Rodnight, R. *Clinical Psychopharmacology*. Lea and Febiger, Philadelphia, 1968.

Shuster, L. Repression and De-Repression of Enzyme Synthesis as a Possible Explanation of Some Aspects of Drug Action. *Nature*, 1961, **189**, 314–315.

Singh, S. D., and Manocha, S. N. The Interaction of Drug Effects with Drive Level and Habit Strength. *Psychopharmacologia*, 1966, **9**, 205–209.

Slanger, S. L., and Miller, N. E. Pharmacological Tests for the Function of Hypothalamic Norepinephrine in Eating Behavior. *Physiology and Behavior*, 1969, **4**, 543–552.

Slater, S. V., and Leavy, A. The Effect of Inhaling a 35 per cent CO_2 and 65 per cent Mixture Upon Anxiety Level in Neurotic Patients. *Behavior and Research Therapy*, 1966, **4**, 309–316.

Smith, C. B. Neurotransmitters and the Narcotic Analgesics. In *Chemical and Biological Aspects of Drug Dependence*. S. U. Mulé and H. Brill (Eds.). CRC Press, Cleveland, 1972, pp. 495–504.

Smyth, D. H. Alimentary Absorption of Drugs: Physiological Considerations. In *Absorption and Distribution of Drugs*. T. B. Binns (Ed.). Williams and Wilkins, Baltimore, 1964, pp. 1–15.

Snyder, S. H., Axelrod, J., and Zweig, M. Circadian Rhythm in the Serotonin Content of the Rat Pineal Gland: Regulating Factors. *Journal of Pharmacology and Experimental Therapeutics*, 1967, **158**, 206–213.

Snyder, S. H., Zweig, N., Axelrod, J., and Fisher, J. E. Control of the Circadian Rhythm in Serotonin Content of the Rat Pineal Gland. *Proceedings of the National Academy of Sciences*, 1965, **53**, 301–305.

Sotelo, C. General Features of the Synaptic Organization in the Central Nervous System. In *Chemistry and Brain Development*. R. Paoletti and A. N. Dawison (Eds.). Plenum Press, New York, 1971.

Spector, S., Milman, K., and Sjoerdsma, A. Evidence for the Rapid Turnover of Norepinephrine in the Rat Heart and Brain. *Proceedings of the Society for Experimental Biology and Medicine*, 1962, **111**, 79–80.

Spehlmann, R. Acetylcholine and Prostigmine Electrophoresis at Visual Cortex Neurons. *Journal of Neurophysiology*, 1963, **26**, 127–139.

Spooner, C. E., Winters, W. D., and Mandell, A. J. DL-Norepinephrine-7-H^3 Uptake, Water Content, and Thiocyanate Space in the Brain during Maturation. *Federation Proceedings*, 1966, **25**, 451.

Starzl, T. E., Taylor, C. W., and Magoun, H. W. Ascending Conduction in Reticular Activating System with Special Reference to the Diencephalon. *Journal of Neurophysiology*, 1951, **14**, 461–496.

Stein, L. Anticholinergic Drugs and Central Control of Thirst. *Science*, 1963, **139**, 46–48.

Stein, L., and Seifter, J. Muscarinic Synapses in the Hypothalamus. *American Journal of Physiology*, 1962, **202**, 751–756.

Stein, L., and Wise, C. D. Possible Aetiology of Schizophrenia: Progressive Damage to the Noradrenergic Reward System by 6-OH-Dopamine. *Science*, 1971, **171**, 1032–1033.

Stephenson, R. P. A Modification of Receptor Theory. *British Journal of Pharmacology*, 1956, **11**, 379–393.

Stevens, C. F. *Neurophysiology: A Primer*. John Wiley, New York, 1966.

Stockley, I. H. Basic Principles of Drug Interaction. *Chemistry in Britain*, 1972, **8**, 114–118.

Stoll, W. A. Lysergsäure-diäthyl-amid ein phantastikum aus Mutter Korngruppe. *Schweizer Archives Neurologie und psychiatrie*, 1947, **60**, 279–323.

Sturman, J. A., and Smith, M. J. H. The Binding of Salicylates to Plasma Protein in Different Species. *Journal of Pharmacy and Pharmacology*, 1967, **19**, 621–623.

Szeinberg, A., and Sheba, Ch. Pharmacogenetics. *Israel Journal of Medical Sciences*, 1968, **4**, 488–493.

Tagliamonte, A., Tagliamonte, P., and Gessa, G. L. Reversal of Pargyline-Induced Inhibition of Sexual Behavior in Male Rats by *p*-Chlorophenylalanine. *Nature*, 1971, **230**, 244–245.

Tagliamonte, A., Tagliamonte, P., Gessa, G. L., and Brodie, B. B. Compulsive Sexual Behavior Induced by *p*-Chlorophenylalanine in Normal and Adrenalectomized Male Rats. *Science*, 1969, **166**, 1433–1435.

Tapp, J. T., Zimmermann, R. S., and D'Encurnaçao, P. S. Intercorrelational Analysis of Some Common Measures of Rat Activity. *Psychological Reports*, 1968, **23**, 1047–1056.

Teitelbaum, P., and Stellar, E. Recovery from the Failure to Eat Produced by Hypothalamic Lesions. *Science*, 1954, **120**, 894–895.

Terrace, H. S. Errorless Discrimination Learning in the Pigeon: Effects of Chlorpromazine and Imipramine. *Science*, 1963, **140**, 318–319.

Thoenen, H. Chemical Sympathectomy: A New Tool in the Investigation of the Physiology and Pharmacology of peripheral and Central Adrenergic Neurons. In *Perspectives in Neuropharmacology*. S. H. Snyder (Ed.). Oxford University Press, New York, 1972, pp. 301–338.

Thompson, T., and Schuster, C. R. *Behavioral Pharmacology*. Prentice-Hall, Englewood Cliffs, N. J., 1968.

Thompson, W. R., and Grusec, J. E. Studies of Early Experience. In *Carmichael's Manual of Child Psychology*. T. Mussen (Ed.). John Wiley, New York, 1970.

Tilson, H. A., and Sparber, S. B. Differences in Tolerance to Mescaline Produced by Peripheral and Direct Central Administration. *Psychopharmacologia*, 1971, **19**, 313–323.

Tobias, J. M., Lipton, M. A., and Lepinat, A. A. Effect of Anesthetics and Convulsants on Brain Acetylcholine Content. *Proceedings of the Society for Experimental Biology and Medicine*, 1946, **61**, 51–54.

Toman, J. E. P. Neurotropic Drugs. In *Neurochemistry*. K. A. C. Elliott, I. H. Page, and J. H. Quastel (Eds.). Charles C Thomas, Springfield, Ill., 1962, pp. 728–765.

Toner, P. G., and Carr, K. E. *Cell Structure*. Williams and Wilkins, Baltimore, 1968.

Travell, J. The Influence of the Hydrogen Ion Concentration on the Absorption of Alkaloids from the Stomach. *Journal of Pharmacology and Experimental Therapeutics*, 1940, **69**, 21–33.

Udenfriend, S., and Creveling, C. R. Localization of Dopamine-β-oxidase in Brain. *Journal of Neurochemistry*, 1959, **4**, 350–352.

Udenfriend, S., Bogdanski, D. F., and Weissband, H. Biochemistry and Metabolism of Serotonin as it Relates to the Nervous System. In *Metabolism of the Nervous System*. D. Richter (Ed.). Pergamon Press, Oxford, 1957, pp. 566–577.

Vernier, V. G., Boren, J. J., Knapp, P. G., and Malis, J. L. The Effect of Drugs on Self-Determined Intercranial Aversive Thresholds. *American Journal of Medical Science*, 1961, **242**, 651–653.

Vesell, E. S. Genetic and Environmental Factors Affecting Hexobarbital Metabolism in Mice. *Annals of the New York Academy of Sciences*, 1968, **151**, 900–912.

Vogt, M. Concentration of Sympathin in Different Parts of the Central Nervous System under Normal Conditions and after the Administration of Drugs. *Journal of Physiology*, 1954, **123**, 451–481.

Volle, R. L. Cholinomimetic Drugs, In *Drill's Pharmacology in Medicine*. J. R. Dipalma (Ed.). McGraw-Hill, New York, 1971.

von Euler, U. S. A Specific Sympathomimetic Ergone in Adrenergic Nerve Fibres (Sympathin) and its Relations to Adrenaline and Noradrenaline. *Acta Physiologica Scandinavica*, 1946, **12**, 73–97.

van Rossum, J. M. The Significance of Dopamine-Receptor Blockade for the Mechanism of Action of Neuroleptic Drugs. *Archives Internationales de Pharmacodyanmics et de Thérapie*, 1966, **160**, 492–494.

van Rossum, J. M., and Ariens, E. J. Receptor-Reserve and Threshold Phenomena. *Archives Internationales de Pharmacodynamics et de Thérapie*, 1962, **136**, 385–413.

Waelsch, H. Blood-Brain Barrier and Gas Exchange. In *Biochemistry of the Developing Nervous System*. H. Waelsch (Ed.). Academic Press, New York, 1955.

Wallace, G. B., and Brodie, B. B. The Distribution of Iodide, Thiocyanate, Bromide and Chloride in the Central Nervous System and Spinal Fluid. *Journal of Pharmacology and Experimental Therapeutics*, 1939, **65**, 220–226.

Walters, G. C., and Abel, E. L. Passive Avoidance Learning in Rats, Gerbils, and Hamsters. *Psychonomic Science*, 1971, **22**, 269–270.

Wang, R. I. H., Hasegarva, A. T., Peters, N. J., and Rimin, A. Amphetamine Toxicity in Isolated and Aggregated Mice. *Psychopharmacologia*, 1969, **15**, 102–108.

Warner, G. F., Dobson, E. L., Pace, N., Johnston, M. E., and Finney, C. R. Studies of Human Peripheral Blood Flow: The Effect of Injection Volume on the Intramuscular Radiosodium Clearance Rate. *Ciruclation*, 1953, **8**, 732–734.

Watanabe, H. The Development of Tolerance to and of Physical Dependence on Morphine Following Intraventricular Injection in the Rat. *Japanese Journal of Pharmacology*, 1971, **21**, 383–391.

Weaver, L. C., and Kerley, T. L. Strain Difference in Response of Mice to d-Amphetamine. *Journal of Pharmacology and Experimental Therapeutics*, 1962, **135**, 240–244.

Weil-Malherbe, H., and Bone, A. D. Intracellular Distribution of Catecholamines in the Brain. *Nature*, 1957, **180**, 1050–1051.

Weil-Malherbe, H., Whitbey, L. G., and Axelrod, J. The Blood Brain Barrier for Catecholamines in Different Regions of the Brain. In *Regional Neurochemistry*. S. S. Kety and J. Elkes (Eds.). Pergamon Press, New York, 1961, pp. 284–291.

Weiskrantz, L., and Wilson, L. The Effects of Reserpine on Emotional Behavior of Normal and Brain-Operated Monkeys. *Annals of the New York Academy of Sciences*, 1955, **61**, 36–55.

Werman, R. Criteria for Identification of a Central Nervous System Transmitter. *Comparative Biochemistry and Physiology*, 1966, **18**, 745–766.

Whalen, R. E., and Luttge, W. G. p-Chlorophenylalanine Methyl Ester: An Aphrodisiac? *Science*, 1970, **169**, 1000–1001.

Wikler, A. Adaptive Behavior in Long-surviving Dogs Without Neocortex. *Archives of Neurology and Psychiatry*, 1950, **64**, 29–41.

Wikler, A. Theories Related to Physical Dependence. In *Chemical and Biological Aspects of Drug Dependence*. S. J. Mulé and H. Brill (Eds.). CRC Press, Cleveland, 1972, pp. 359–377.

Wilder, J. The Law of Initial Value in Neurology and Psychiatry. Facts and Problems. *Journal of Nervous and Mental Disease*, 1957, **125**, 73–86.

Williams, R. T. *Biochemical Individuality. The Basis for the Genototrophic Concept*. John Wiley, New York, 1956.

Williams, R. T. Species Variations in Drug Biotransformations. In *Fundamentals of Drug Metabolism and Drug Disposition*. B. N. LaDu, H. G. Mandel, and E. L. Way (Eds.). Williams and Wilkins, Baltimore, 1971, pp. 187–205.

Winter, C. A., and Flataker, L. Cage Design as a Factor Influencing Acute Toxicity of Respiratory Depressant Drugs in Rats. *Toxicology and Applied Pharmacology*, 1962, **4**, 650–655.

Wisham, L. H., Yalow, R. S., and Freund, A. J. Consistency of Clearance of Radioactive Sodium from Human Muscle. *American Heart Journal*, 1951, **41**, 810–818.

Wolf, H. H., Swinyard, E. A., and Clark, L. D. The Differential Effects of Chlorpromazine and Pentobarbital on Two Forms of Conditioned Avoidance Behavior in *Peromyscus Maniculatus Gracilis*. *Psychopharmacologia*, 1962, **3**, 438–448.

Wolpe, J. *Psychotherapy by Reciprocal Inhibition*. Stanford University Press, Stanford, 1958.

Wooley, D. W., and Gommi, B. W. Serotonin Receptors. IV. Specific Deficiency of Receptors in Galactose Poisoning and its Possible Relationship to the Idiocy of Galactosemia. *Proceedings of the National Academy of Sciences*, 1962, **52**, 14.

Wooley, D. W., and Gommi, B. W. Serotonin Receptors: V, Selective Destruction by Neuramindase Plus EDTA and Reactivation with Tissue Lipids. *Nature*, 1964, **202**, 1074.

Wurtman, R. J., and Axelrod, J. Daily Rhythmic Changes in Tyrosine Transaminase Activity of the Rat Liver. *Proceedings of the National Academy of Sciences*, 1967, **57**, 1594–1598.

Yaffe, S. J., Krasner, J., and Catz, C. S. Variations in Detoxication Enzymes During Mammalian Development. *Annals of the New York Academy of Sciences*, 1968, **151**, 887–899.

Yamamoto, C. Pharmacologic Studies of Norepinephrine, Acetylcholine and Related Compounds on Neurons in Deiter's Nucleus and the Cerebellum. *Journal of Pharmacology*, 1967, **156**, 39–47.

Yeary, R. A., Benish, R. A., and Finkelstein, M. Acute Toxicity of Drugs in Newborn Animals. *Journal of Pediatrics*, 1966, **69**, 663–667.

Yehuda, S., and Wurtman, R. J. The Effects of D-Amphetamine and Related Drugs on Colonic Temperatures of Rats Kept at Various Ambient Temperature. *Life Sciences*, 1972, **11**, 851–859.

York, D. H. The Inhibitory Actions of Dopamine on Neurones of the Caudate Nucleus. *Brain Research*, 1967, **5**, 263–266.

York, D. H., and McLennan, H. Cholinergic and Dopaminergic Mechanisms in the Caudate Nucleus. *Australian Journal of Experimental Biological Science*, 1967, **45**, 10–15.

Young, J. Z. Growth and Plasticity in the Nervous System. *Proceedings of the Royal Society of Biology*, 1951, **139**, 18–37.

Zweig, M., Snyder, S. H., and Axelrod, J. Evidence for a Non-Retinal Pathway of Light to the Pineal Gland of Newborn Rats. *Proceedings of the National Academy of Sciences*, 1966, **56**, 515–520.

Author Index

Subject Index